The Problem Knee

Second edition

Malcolm F. Macnicol

MBChB, BSc (Hons), FRCS, MCh, FRCS Ed (Orth)
Consultant Orthopaedic Surgeon
(Princess Margaret Rose Orthopaedic Hospital,
Royal Hospital for Sick Children and
Royal Infirmary, Edinburgh) and
Senior Orthopaedic Lecturer, University of Edinburgh, UK

ROH Library
WITHDRAWN

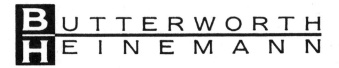

BUTTERWORTH
HEINEMANN

Butterworth-Heinemann
Linacre House, Jordan Hill, Oxford OX2 8DP
A division of Reed Educational and Professional Publishing Ltd

A member of the Reed Elsevier plc group

OXFORD   BOSTON   JOHANNESBURG
MELBOURNE   NEW DELHI   SINGAPORE

First published 1986
Second edition 1995
Paperback edition 1998

© Reed Educational and Professional Publishing Ltd 1995

All rights reserved. No part of this publication
may be reproduced in any material form (including
photocopying or storing in any medium by electronic
means and whether or not transiently or incidentally
to some other use of this publication) without the
written permission of the copyright holder except
in accordance with the provisions of the Copyright,
Designs and Patents Act 1988 or under the terms of a
licence issued by the Copyright Licensing Agency Ltd,
90 Tottenham Court Road, London, England W1P 9HE.
Applications for the copyright holder's written permission
to reproduce any part of this publication should be addressed
to the publishers

British Library Cataloguing in Publication Data
Macnicol, Malcolm F.
  The Problem Knee. - 2 Rev. ed
  I. Title
  616.7

ISBN 0 7506 4044 8

Library of Congress Cataloguing in Publication Data
Macnicol, Malcolm F.
  The Problem Knee / Malcolm F. Macnicol. - 2nd ed.
  p. cm.
  Includes bibliographical references and index.
  ISBN 0 7506 4044 8
  1. Knee-Wounds and injuries. I. Title
  [DNLM: 1. Knee Injuries-diagnosis. 2. Knee Injuries-
  rehabilitation. WE 870 M169p 1995]
  RD561.M33 1995
  617.5'82-dc20
  DNLM/DLC   94-45158
  for Library of Congress   CIP

Composition by Scribe Design, Gillingham, Kent
Printed in Great Britain by The Bath Press plc, Avon

Contents

Preface

The knee is a complex and crucial joint, as easily injured during the daily round as in competitive sports, industrial accidents or collisions. While the causes of acute or chronic knee symptoms are not always apparent, it is to be hoped that, at very least, an informed questioning and examination of the patient or injured athlete will ensure that needless morbidity is avoided. Whether the inextricable mix of synovitis, torn ligament or meniscus, and osteochondral damage can be teased apart may in the end depend upon the experience and investigative skills of the surgeon; but assuredly a lack of cooperation and free communication with colleagues in other disciplines will retard both the speed and successes of treatment.

This short book emphasises the basic principles in managing a 'problem knee'. The inter-relationship between soft tissue and skeletal injuries is acknowledged, but in the interests of a simplified and rational approach, separate chapters deal with the various components of the joint. Details about surgical technique have been expressly avoided, in part because these can only be learnt effectively in the operating theatre. Since the first edition was published, magnetic resonance imaging and dynamic computerised tomography have been widely introduced. Yet these investigations do not rule out the importance of history taking, careful and standardised physical examination, and conventional radiography. The unconditional use of diagnostic arthroscopy and scanning cannot be condoned, and the expense of unnecessary investigation and surgical intervention will become an increasing burden in the future if the basic clinical assessment is not undertaken carefully.

Operative intervention for patellar pain is much less frequently advised than in the past, and there remains concern about defining maltracking and the subtleties of patellar instability. Cruciate ligament reconstruction, on the other hand, is much more commonly undertaken, and generally with good effect. In selected cases, meniscal repair and osteochondral grafting are appropriate, and after all forms of surgery, a more rapid rehabilitation is espoused.

The text now incorporates references to important papers about the knee, and expands upon sports injury in childhood, the management of ligament tears and the importance of graduated exercise during the recovery period. Systemic conditions are described as they relate to the knee in younger individuals, but degenerative conditions are excluded.

The first edition of *The Problem Knee* appealed particularly to physiotherapists, coaches, family doctors and casualty officers. It is to be hoped that this edition will also provide a basic approach to knee problems in the younger patient for those in orthopaedic surgical practice.

Acknowledgements

I wish to record my thanks to Miss Pamela Copeland for her help in all stages of preparing and typing the manuscript of the second edition. Additional photography has been provided by Michael Devlin, further illustrations drawn by Ian Lennox and suggestions from Martin Rennison included in Chapter 10. My approach to the management of the problem knee has been much influenced by discussion and cooperation with colleagues over the years, and I wish to thank them for their promptings that a second edition be published.

1

The mechanism and presentation of injuries to the knee

INTRODUCTION – HISTORY – ANATOMY – CLINICAL
PRESENTATION

INTRODUCTION

The knee is designed for rapid and complex movements; at the same time,
it is usually encumbered with the weight of the body. These two require-
ments, speed and strength, place stresses upon the joint which may in turn
produce symptoms. Another characteristic is the exposed position of the
knee which makes it vulnerable in many occupations and sports. The
combination of this vulnerability to injury and its underlying sophistica-
tion must be kept in mind not simply when identifying the mechanism of
injuries to the knee but also when planning a return to normal activities,
let alone to strenuous forms of work or to athletics.

There are four principal groups who may present with symptoms from
the knee. First, there are those who are relatively unfit in whom a mild
congenital weakness makes the knee slightly unstable and subsequently
symptomatic. Secondly, there is the athletic individual who subjects his
knees to repetitive stress or considerable loads, with subsequent fatigue of
not only the soft tissues but also the bony structures of the femur, tibia and
patella. There is a third group of otherwise normal subjects whose knees
are subjected to a sudden high-velocity collision or fall which exceeds the
strength of the components of the knee, for example, those involved in
motorcycle accidents. Finally, there is a small number of individuals in
whom injuries to the knee seem inextricably and frustratingly linked with
a personality problem or neurosis.

The knee joint is supported by its capsule, the ligaments and surrounding muscles, with assistance from the menisci and the patellofemoral joint.
The configuration of the femoral and tibial articular surfaces is principally
concerned with weightbearing and the relatively unconstrained hinging that
occurs between them is designed for speed of movement. The
patellofemoral joint improves the efficiency of the quadriceps muscle, and
hence the strength of knee extension. Regrettably, as with the tibiofemoral
articulation, the patellofemoral joint is prone to instability, and to stresses

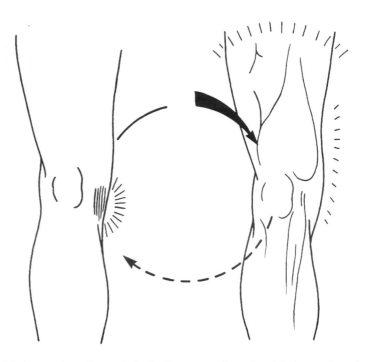

Figure 1.1 *A protective reflex arc links the ligaments and muscles of the knee; when a ligament, such as the medial collateral is stretched, impulses are referred by the afferent nerves to the spinal cord. Efferent nerves then transmit the signal to the muscles which contract appropriately, thus enhancing the stabilizing of the knee. Proprioception is also afforded by other structures in the knee (see Table 5.1)*

that produce symptoms in the vicinity of that specialized sesamoid bone, the patella.

The biological trade-off between mobility and stability is largely governed by the proprioceptive arc formed by the ligaments and their companion muscles (Figure 1.1). A break in this feedback loop not only reduces function but imperils long-term recovery since the balance between stability and a free range of movement is easily upset.

HISTORY

Obtaining a clear history of the events that lead to an injury of the knee is difficult, but always important. Indeed, a careful history is often of greater diagnostic value than clinical examination or subsequent investigations. Unfortunately memory of events is often blurred by the speed with which many injuries occur, and in some cases by the time which has elapsed before diagnosis is requested. Apart from the rare occasions when a patient conceals the nature of an injury, or its circumstances if litigation complicates the issue, a reasonably accurate statement can usually be produced if the correct questions are asked.

Since the knee joint can be stressed in any direction, the mechanism of injury may involve valgus or varus forces, excessive extension or flexion,

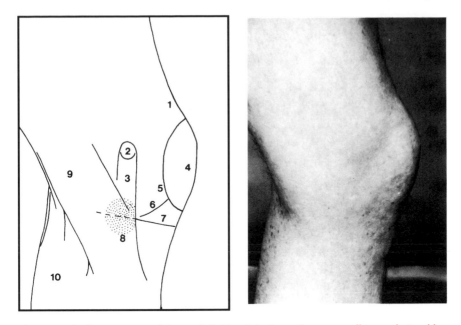

Figure 1.2 Surface anatomy of the medial side of the knee: [1, suprapatellar pouch; 2, adductor tubercle; 3, medial (tibial) collateral ligament; 4, patella; 5, parapatellar synovium; 6, anterior edge of the medial femoral condyle; 7, medial joint line (defining the peripheral rim of the medial meniscus); 8, 'no man's land' where the medial ligament and medial meniscus overlap; 9, the 'pes anserinus' (sartorius, gracilis and semitendinosus tendons); 10, semimembranosus and medial head of the gastrocnemius muscles].

and extremes of internal and external rotation. Violent anterior or posterior movement of the tibia in relation to the femur, or axially directed forces, are not uncommon, many soft-tissue injuries and fractures occurring as a result of a combination of these forces. As if that were not enough, malfunction of the patellofemoral joint may complicate and confuse the picture further; hence, it is important to understand as much about the mechanism of injury as possible, a task made difficult by the rapidity of many accidents.

ANATOMY

A knowledge of the anatomy of the knee is essential if the extent of the structural damage is to be assessed accurately. Certain landmarks of surface anatomy are palpable, including the medial and lateral joint lines and lateral ligaments and the extent of the suprapatellar pouch (Figures 1.2a,b and 1.3a,b). Additional bony landmarks include the tibial tuberosity, which may be laterally placed, Gerdy's tubercle and a bony prominence in relation to the superolateral pole of the patella produced by a secondary ossification centre. The position of the femoral condyles, the infrapatellar fat pad, the common peroneal nerve and the infrapatellar branch of the saphenous nerve should also be appreciated (see Figure 2.5).

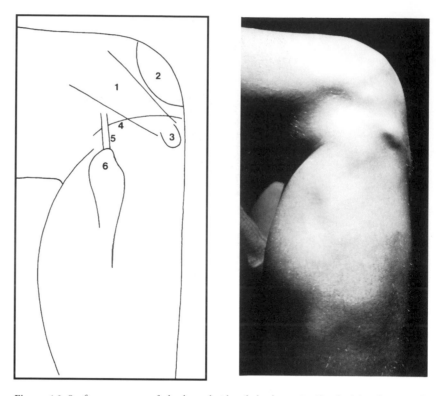

Figure 1.3 *Surface anatomy of the lateral side of the knee: [1, iliotibial band; 2, patella; 3, Gerdy's tubercle where part of the band inserts into the tibia; 4, lateral joint line (defining the peripheral rim of the lateral mensicus); 5, lateral (fibular) collateral ligament; 6, fibular head].*

Medial side of the knee

Figure 1.4 shows the structures that overlie the medial side of the knee. These may be injured in sequential fashion by a valgus force applied to the leg, and thus the medial capsule and its important posteromedial corner, the medial collateral ligament, the medial meniscus, the posterior capsule, the anterior cruciate ligament and the patellar retinaculum may all be partially or completely torn. Major violence may also tear the posterior cruciate ligament, in which case a knee dislocation becomes likely, and will involve the more distant structures such as the lateral meniscus and the pes anserinus (the sartorius, gracilis and semitendinosus muscles over the medial aspect of the knee).

Rotational stresses usually coexist with the valgus force and will determine to a great extent the involvement of the various components of the medal side of the knee. Some structures may rupture completely, whereas others may remain 'in continuity' but weakened. Fractures involving articular surfaces or ligament attachments may occur instead, particularly in the child or the elderly patient where the strength of the cancellous bone is less than that of connective tissue making up the ligaments.

Lateral side of the knee

A similar cascade of injuries may occur when a varus force is applied to the knee (Figure 1.5). The structures involved include the fibular (lateral)

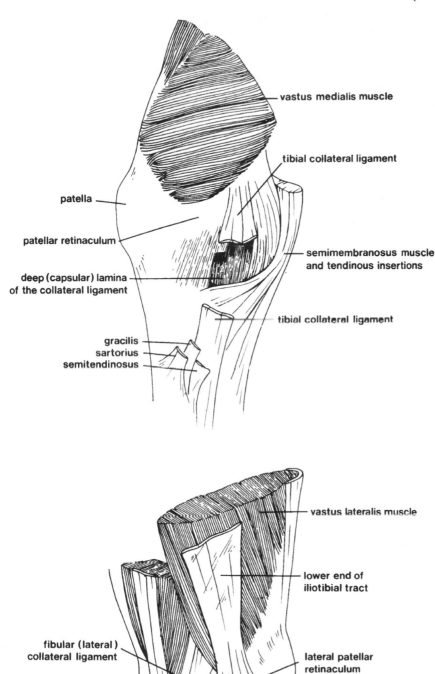

vastus medialis muscle

tibial collateral ligament

patella

patellar retinaculum

semimembranosus muscle
and tendinous insertions

deep (capsular) lamina
of the collateral ligament

tibial collateral ligament

gracilis
sartorius
semitendinosus

Figure 1.4 *Soft-tissue anatomy of the medial side of the knee*

vastus lateralis muscle

lower end of
iliotibial tract

fibular (lateral)
collateral ligament

lateral patellar
retinaculum

biceps tendon

patella

head of fibula

Figure 1.5 *Soft-tissue anatomy of the lateral side of the knee*

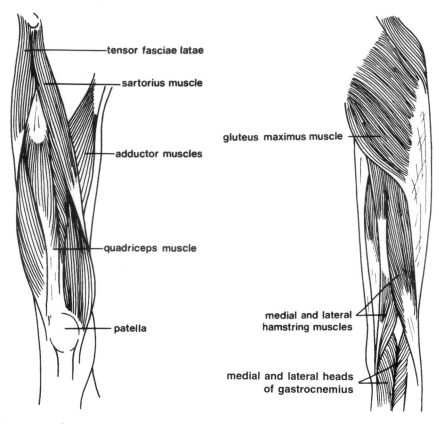

Figure 1.6 *The anterior thigh muscles*

Figure 1.7 *The posterior thigh and superficial calf muscles*

collateral ligament, the iliotibial band, the arcuate complex, the lateral meniscus, the posterior cruciate ligament, the posterior capsule, the anterior cruciate ligament, the biceps tendon, the peroneal nerve, the popliteus tendon and the medial meniscus.

Once again, various patterns of damage are possible within these tissues. However, a more precise assessment of the extent of these soft-tissue injuries will be presented in the chapters dealing with the clinical examination and problems of the menisci, ligaments and patellofemoral joint.

Finally, the muscles acting across the knee may be injured and a knowledge of their anatomy is essential. Although the importance of the quadriceps muscle (Figure 1.6) is appreciated by those who treat injuries of the knee, significant morbidity may also follow injury to the gluteus maximus and the iliotibial tract, to the hamstring muscles and the medial and lateral heads of the gastrocnemius muscle in the calf (Figures 1.7 and 1.8).

CLINICAL PRESENTATION

When taking a history, specific questions should be asked about:

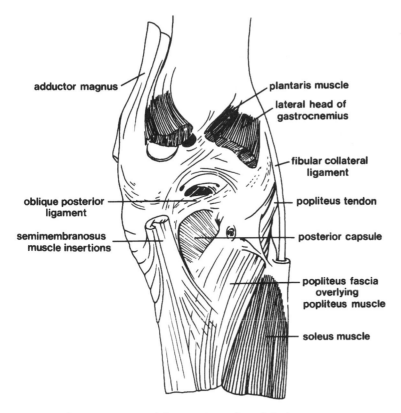

Figure 1.8 Soft-tissue anatomy of the posterior surface of the knee

- Pain
- Loss of the normal range of movement
- Swelling
- Abnormal mobility (instability)

Pain

Pain is not often well localized (Figure 1.9), although an associated tenderness may well be. However, secondary but mild injuries to other structures may even make the relevance of the apparently localized tenderness uncertain, such as patellar subluxation producing pain and tenderness over the medial side of the knee, suggesting medial ligamentous or meniscal damage; or tears in one meniscus referring symptoms, and even signs, to the contralateral compartment of the knee. Nevertheless, it is important to describe pain as precisely as possible, noting *site, periodicity, precipitating factors* and any *referral* of the discomfort.

Loss of movement

Loss of movement is usually described by the patient as a feeling of stiffness, or as a 'block' to the full range of knee extension or flexion. Both

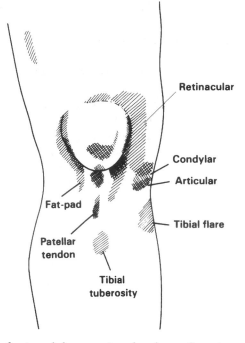

Figure 1.9 *The referral of pain and the perception of tenderness from the patellofemoral joint is confusing*

these forms of restriction may be painful, and usually there is a limp or some alteration in gait. Rotation of the tibia below the femur is also impaired.

Stiffness indicates that the periphery and possibly also the articular surfaces of the joint are abnormal. This increased resistance to movement throughout the range of flexion is characteristic of an inflammatory condition, with or without a significant effusion present. A more unyielding form of stiffness develops in time, particularly if muscle and soft-tissue contractures occur, or if the osteoarthritic process alters articular surfaces markedly.

Locking

True locking may be intermittent or persistent. A relatively painless block to extension, or flexion deformity, and the loss of flexion resulting from chronic arthritis should be distinguished from the springy and often exquisitely painful block produced by a torn meniscus or loose body. Other structures may cause a form of locking of the knee, and particularly in children this may lead to an erroneous diagnosis of meniscal tear. True locking may also occur if a cruciate stump is present in the knee or if there is any other impingement that affects the normally free range of knee excursion.

The circumstances that cause the knee to feel stiff or locked should also be identified. An inflammatory process will cause the joint to feel stiff after a night's sleep or after a period of prolonged sitting, classically after a car journey or in a cinema or waiting room. Locking tends to be noticed during activity more than at rest, although it may be accompanied by a sense of stiffness after the knee has been kept in flexion whether during crouching or sitting. Certain unguarded movements, particularly twisting on the flexed knee, are not only potent causes of meniscal tears, but also produce further episodes of locking, and a resultant extension of the tear (Figure 1.10).

Trillat (1962) described the progression of a vertical tear which may either proceed through the central portion of the meniscus, forming a bucket handle tear, or may rupture through the posterior horn, producing a flap. The bucket handle may tear across centrally, resulting in various sizes of anterior and posterior flaps, or may rupture through the anterior horn. Locking may then become intermittent or cease, although the patient may feel something moving within the knee or protruding at the joint line. Dandy (1990) has also described his experience with different meniscal tears, and offers an alternative classification, although the nature of the lesions is basically the same.

The presence of a pathological meniscus usually causes some loss of passive movement, even in the chronic stages. However, minor peripheral splits may heal with time, and smaller flaps and tags may be thinned out to the extent that they cease to trouble the patient. The horizontal cleavage lesions, and some oblique degenerative tears, may also become asymptomatic so that their excision is less commonly practised than before (Noble and Hamblen, 1975; Noble and Erat, 1980). It can also be surprising to find the occasional case of completely displaced bucket handle tear in a patient with atypical or minimal symptoms. Certain types of work or sport will, of course, highlight any restriction, and thus an athlete or labourer will be unable to tolerate functional deficiencies which may be accepted by a sedentary worker.

Swelling

A rapid swelling of the knee after injury is usually noted quite accurately by the patient, whereas more gradual swelling may be misinterpreted with regard to both the site and extent of the swelling. An acute swelling almost always means that bleeding has occurred into the joint, and this haemarthrosis is a sign that a vascular structure has been torn. Synovial and ligament tears will therefore produce a haemarthrosis, as will an intra-articular fracture. These aspects are dealt with more fully in the chapters concerned with examination and investigation of the injured knee.

More gradual swelling suggests that an effusion has occurred, and this may not be noted as significant by the patient, or may only be observed the following day after an injury. Meniscal tears and sprains of the knee produce effusions, since they both trigger off a synovitis. The importance of assessing synovial fluid in post-traumatic conditions and in various arthropathies is dealt with in Chapter 9.

An effusion will fill the synovial cavity of the knee including the suprapatellar pouch (see Plate 28) and the extent of the swelling may confuse the injured person. Other, more discrete swellings can also affect the knee (see Plates 29 and 30) and their appearance is more insidious, but may also, as with an effusion, prove to be intermittent.

(a)

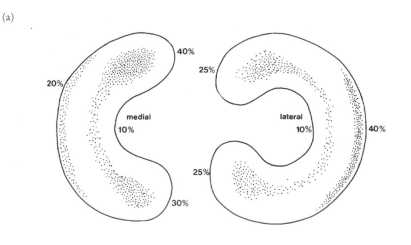

(b)

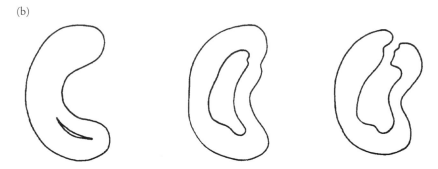

progression of a vertical tear to a bucket handle lesion and then a pedunculated tag

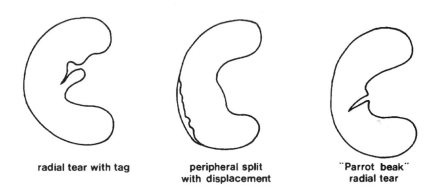

| radial tear with tag | peripheral split with displacement | "Parrot beak" radial tear |

Figure 1.10 (a) the approximate incidence of traumatic tears at various sites in both menisci. (b) the upper three diagrams show the typical progression of a posterior, vertical meniscal tear to a 'bucket handle' lesion and eventually to a pedunculated tag (left to right); the lower three diagrams show an inner rim tag, a peripheral split causing slight meniscal displacement and a 'parrot beak' radial tear (from left to right).

Classically, a mild effusion occurs after twisting injuries of the knee if a low-grade synovitis or meniscal tear is chronically present. The effusion disappears after the knee has been rested and then reappears after further stress. Detection of this fluid is an important part of the examination and the swelling can be graded into minor, moderate or severe (tense). The physiotherapist or doctor can use the presence or absence of an effusion after exercise as a monitor of the progress of a patient, the precipitation of fluid suggesting that the responsible activity is too great for the knee to contend with at that stage of recovery. If a synovitis with its associated effusion becomes established, it can prove difficult to treat and there may be a place for anti-inflammatory agents in this instance. Arthroscopy and irrigation of the joint may also cause an effusion to disappear.

If a patient states that his knee regularly becomes swollen, but no fluid or discrete swelling can be found on the day of examination, it is often useful to request the patient to return on a day when the swelling is apparent. The nature and site of such a swelling is of great diagnostic value and the importance of describing this carefully cannot be overstated.

Instability

Direct violence to the knee may make the joint incompetent when bearing the weight of the body, particularly when angulatory and rotational stresses are also being applied to the leg. Instability of this sort can be very troublesome, and the knee may give way in a most unexpected and dangerous fashion. Anterolateral instability, where the convex lateral tibial condyle and lateral meniscus sublux under the lateral femoral condyle, clinically causes a feeling of two knuckles rubbing over each other, and a painful buckling results (see Chapter 5).

Although ligament tears in various combinations are responsible for many forms of quite gross instability, the knee may also yield under load if the patella subluxes laterally or if the axis of knee movement is altered by the presence of a meniscal lesion or a loose body. Additional causes of buckling of the knee include chronic weakness of the quadriceps muscle, or a reflex inhibition of its contraction owing to some obstructing or painful lesion in the joint. Usually this functional instability occurs during manoeuvres such as climbing ladders or negotiating rough ground, when the quadriceps mechanism is under greater load. However, instability secondary to weakness may occur suddenly and for no apparent reason, such that the patient falls to the ground.

Personality of the individual

The significance of the cardinal symptoms – pain, loss of movement and instability – will be influenced by the demands placed upon the knee by the individual, and by his personality and expectations of physical fitness. Athletes will tolerate poorly a relatively minor abnormality which a less active person may accept perfectly readily. A clicking sensation in the joint or patellofemoral crepitus are common enough features, but may provoke great anxiety in the introspective individual. One person may shrug off a symptom, whereas for another the persistence of a minor disability may

Table 1.1 Common causes of knee symptoms related to the age and sex of the patient

Age (years)	Sex	
	Female	*Male*
5–10	Discoid lateral meniscus Synovitis or arthropathy Fractures Patellar instability Soft-tissue tumours	Discoid lateral meniscus Synovitis, arthropathy, haemophilia Fractures Soft tissue tumours
10–20	Patellar instability Patellar pain (?stress) Ligament rupture Osteochondritis dissecans Fracture Arthropathy	Osteochondritis dissecans Meniscal tears Osteochondroses Patellar instability Fracture Ligament rupture Arthropathy
20–30	Patellar instability Cystic lateral meniscus Arthropathy Ligament rupture Meniscal tear	Meniscal tear Ligament rupture Fracture Arthropathy Cystic lateral meniscus
30+	The problems detailed above, often superimposed upon increasing degenerative changes	

preoccupy the mind. During adolescence, pains in the knee may prove very troublesome for not only the patient but also the parents, and eventually the doctor and physiotherapist. There may come a time, particularly when pain is not associated with any obvious mechanical problem, when the patient is asked to 'live with the pain'.

Such counsel is often hard to give, and even harder to accept. But if clinical examination, basic medical investigations, radiographs, magnetic resonance imaging, arthroscopy and possibly a bone scan have ruled out significant pathology, advice that the patient will have to endure the symptoms is often accepted if there has been a frank explanation of the position (Sandow and Goodfellow, 1985). In the adolescent, some hope should be entertained that the condition may resolve at the end of the skeletal growth or in early adult life, and a change in training methods or sports competition may reduce the frequency of symptoms.

Age-related symptoms

The age group of the patients is therefore important and will also indicate likely causes for the symptoms (Table 1.1). In children, problems usually relate to patellar malalignment syndromes, congenital abnormalities, such as a discoid lateral meniscus, stress or avulsion fractures, and arthropathies secondary to juvenile chronic arthritis or haemophilia. Meniscal tears are relatively rare, and other causes of apparent knee locking should be considered, including osteochondritis dissecans.

After puberty, girls are prone to patellar pain, and this may be related to compression stresses or instability of the knee cap secondary to torsional abnormalities of the legs, to ligament laxity and to a growth spurt. The source of the symptoms may be so puzzling and inextricably linked with emotional factors that the surgeon may do more harm than good if he operates (see Figure 4.13).

In juvenile athletes, patellar tracking, an apophysitis, a discoid meniscus or osteochondritis dissecans may be responsible for the symptoms. Ligament injuries are relatively rare but stress fractures are not. The possibility of significant but unrelated pathology such as infection or neoplasia must always be entertained. Meniscal tears become more frequent in later adolescence, and traumatic synovitis or a traction apophysitis such as Osgood–Schlatter's disease can be troublesome.

Lastly, in the 'mature' athlete, between the ages of 20 and 70 years these days, ligament sprains and ruptures, synovial fringe and fatpad lesions, and osteoarthritis must be added to the list of possible diagnoses.

The ensuing chapters will outline the approach to a knee injury, whether obtained during sport or after an accident. Many associated conditions have to be considered, and both the patient and therapist must accept that many injuries will not result in a complete cure. Early, and appropriate, treatment should, however, speed recovery and lessen the risk of long-standing complications.

References

Dandy, D.J. (1990) Arthroscopic anatomy of symptomatic meniscal lesions. *J. Bone Joint Surg.*, **72B**, 628–631

Noble, J.N. and Erat, K. (1980). In defence of the meniscus : a prospective study of 200 meniscectomy patients. *J. Bone Joint Surg.*, **62B**, 7–11

Noble, J.N. and Hamblen, D.L. (1975) The pathology of the degenerate meniscus lesion. *J. Bone Joint Surg.*, **57B**, 180–186

Sandow, M.J. and Goodfellow, J.W. (1985) The natural history of anterior knee pain in adolescents. *J. Bone Joint Surg.*, **67B**, 36–39

Trillat, A. (1962) Lésions traumatique du ménisque interne du genu Classement anatomique et diagnostic clinique. *Rev. Clin. Orthop.*, **48**, 551–563

2
Methods of clinical examination

THE ROUTINE – INSPECTION – PALPATION – MOVEMENT

Careful examination of the knee is essential before enlisting additional tests or arranging an arthroscopy. The history very often suggests the diagnosis. If the physical features are elicited precisely, the diagnosis may be clinched. Attention to the details of examination may also save the patient an unnecessary number of investigations, and should allow the examiner to feel reasonably confident about the form of treatment which is likely to succeed.

THE ROUTINE

It is always helpful to follow a routine when taking a history or conducting an examination. At the beginning, determine if the dynamic tests of *walking, squatting* and '*duck waddling*' should be requested before or after examination of the patient on the couch. A limp may be caused by symptoms in the knee or weakness, but may also mean that an abnormality is present in the hip or some other part of the affected leg. Hence, it is important to assess the locomotor system generally, to rule out obvious neurological disease, and to consider medical conditions which may affect knee function. This applies especially to the arthropathies, to certain skeletal dysplasias and to congenital conditions. Particular attention should be paid at this stage to any abnormality of the lumbar spine, hip joint, leg muscles and the ankle and foot.

Abnormalities lower down the leg should be sought, and it is therefore essential that the patient be undressed to the extent that all of both legs can be seen. Valgus and torsional deformities should be noted and may have a bearing upon the source of pain. Therefore the range of hip movement is part of the examination of knee joint, looking in particular for persistence of excessive anteversion. A stiff hip may eventually cause pain in the knee as the latter joint is called upon to rotate and absorb stresses to an increased degree, and leg length inequality may damage the knee.

INSPECTION

Looking at the knee, both from the front and back, is a logical first step in examination. The appearance of the skin, the presence of scars and their

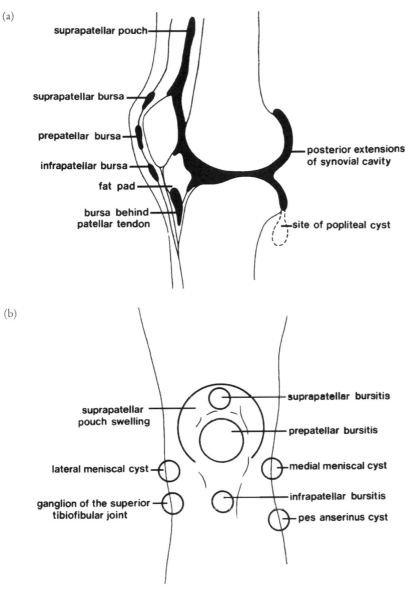

(a)

suprapatellar pouch

suprapatellar bursa

prepatellar bursa

infrapatellar bursa

fat pad

bursa behind patellar tendon

posterior extensions of synovial cavity

site of popliteal cyst

(b)

suprapatellar pouch swelling

lateral meniscal cyst

ganglion of the superior tibiofibular joint

suprapatellar bursitis

prepatellar bursitis

medial meniscal cyst

infrapatellar bursitis

pes anserinus cyst

Figure 2.1 *Cystic swellings around the knee: (a) from the side, (b) from the front*

width, the presence of swellings (Figure 2.1a,b; see Plates 28–31) and the bulk of the quadriceps muscle should be noted. Bruising and ecchymosis may indicate the site and severity of an injury, and if a haemarthrosis has ruptured into the tissues, causing a boggy and ill-defined swelling, then significant ligament and capsular tears should be suspected (Figure 2.2). Other, more discrete, swellings include a lateral meniscus cyst, prepatellar or infrapatellar bursae, popliteal cyst, saphena varix, semimembranosis bursa and Osgood–Schlatter's disease (Figure 2.1; see also Plate 32). Acute injuries may cause a blister, contusion, haematoma, abrasion or laceration.

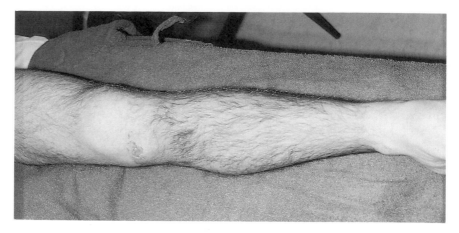

Figure 2.2 *An ecchymosis suggests a significant ligamentous disruption*

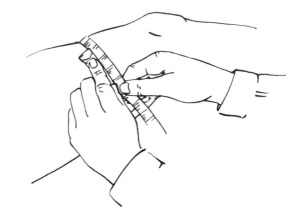

Figure 2.3 *Measurement of the thigh circumference with a tape. The technique is only slightly more accurate than assessing the girth of the thigh by eye*

The chronically injured or inflamed knee will show a classical reversal of contour, in that the thigh muscles gradually waste, while the synovial and capsular envelope enlarges owing to fluid or synovial hypertrophy.

Patella alta may predispose the patient to both patellar pain and lateral subluxation, and the positioning and tracking of the patella should be carefully observed during the course of the clinical examination (see Plates 34 and 35). Linked with any patellar problem is the functioning of the quadriceps muscle and this is most accurately measured by:

- Comparison (from the foot of the bed) with the opposite thigh
- Palpation of the tone of the muscle, particularly vastus medialis, when the patient forcibly extends the knee
- Assessment of thigh circumference using a tape measure at two defined levels, measured above the tibial tuberosity or the upper pole of the patella (Figure 2.3)

A measure of the maximum calf girth in both legs is also recommended, and may indicate whether the leg is generally weaker, rather than the thigh alone.

During the assessment of the knee it is possible to form certain opinions about not merely the physique of the patient but also something of the personality. The response of the patient to questioning and examination often gives vital clues about the manner in which each individual is likely to react to injury, pain and life in general. Small grimaces of pain are often more helpful in deciding where tenderness is located than loud and sometimes unconvincing exclamations from the patient. This is open to misinterpretation, of course, but the interplay between the personality of the patient and the examiner has a greater influence upon the eventual diagnosis than is generally admitted.

At this stage, too, the presence of ligament laxity in other parts of the body and of skin conditions such as psoriasis and eczema should be noted, as these may not only be important aetiologically but may influence recovery after injury. The stigmata of juvenile chronic arthritis and haemophilia are usually clear enough, and in most cases will be documented in the younger patient (see Chapter 9). Nevertheless, an injury or spontaneous symptom in the knee may be the first manifestation of a systemic condition, such that the causes of the various arthropathies, including venereal disease, should be remembered, and general inspection should address these possibilities.

Finally, it is important to stress again the importance of properly viewing the full extent of both the injured and the normal limbs. The contralateral leg is the baseline from which to work, and the knee must be compared to its fellow throughout the examination. Mild abnormalities of function secondary to the build of the patient and the knees are often seen bilaterally and have to be accepted as 'normal' for that individual.

PALPATION

Feeling the temperature and texture of the skin and, as already described, the tone of the quadriceps muscle, augments the picture afforded by the history, the general physique and the appearance of the problem knee. Inflammatory conditions may cause increased warmth and a synovitis produces a thickening of soft tissues. Normal synovium, when picked up between finger and thumb, is barely discernible. However, when engorged and oedematous, a distinct sensation of two slightly rubbery layers moving against each other can be felt. Effusions of varying degree will be encountered. The swollen knee may therefore be principally the result of synovial hypertrophy, or of a haemarthrosis or effusion, or a combination of both.

Swelling

Swellings may be localized as well as generalized, the common sites being over the lateral joint line, in relation to the patella, in the popliteal fossa and arising from muscles such as the semimembranosis and pes anserinus group if the swelling is discrete. Certain swellings are more obvious with

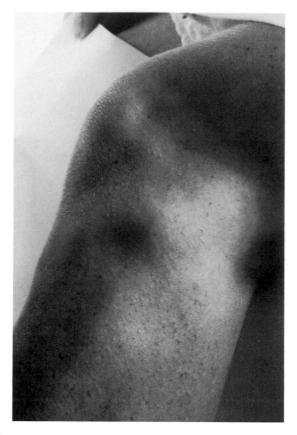

Figure 2.4 *A lateral meniscal cyst made obvious by flexing the knee. A tear of the meniscus is often associated*

the knee straight, particularly effusions and popliteal cysts, whereas others are thrown into relief by flexing the knee (Figure 2.4).

Before assessing the volume of an effusion, it is of value to determine the likely contents of a swelling. Hard lumps which do not transilluminate light are usually bony excrescences. However, they may be partly or completely cartilaginous, such as osteochondromas around the articular margin of the joint and chondral loose bodies. The latter are generally mobile, as their name implies. Synovial chondromatosis (see Plate 48) may also produce firm or hard lumps in the region of the knee as may ectopic calcification.

Ganglia and cysts related to tendons may feel firm, or even hard if they are tense, but they have a habit of varying in size and this should be ascertained from the patient. Cystic swellings are considered traditionally to transilluminate, yet many such cysts around the knee, and classically the lateral meniscal cyst, are deeply placed and loculated, so that convincing transillumination is impossible. Lipomata and certain other soft-tissue lumps may also transmit light in a non-specific manner, and hence this method of assessing a cyst, while useful occasionally, is more often confusing.

Certain swellings may also empty when compressed since a valve effect is commonly present. This accounts for the periodicity of discomfort that characterizes, for example, the popliteal cyst.

Extended knee

With the knee extended, *skin sensation*, the presence of an *effusion* and the *retropatellar* surface can be assessed.

Sensation

Cutaneous nerve distribution is variable (Figure 2.5) but a common problem arises when the infrapatellar branch of the saphenous nerve is accidentally severed during a medial arthrotomy. Furthermore, injuries to the nerve from impaction of the anteromedial aspect of the knee against a car dashboard or other unyielding object are not uncommon. After both a severance or a neuropraxia, the loss of sensation over the front of the knee can be troublesome, especially if a great deal of kneeling is required.

Paraesthesiae may ensue later, and may increase greatly, producing what is termed 'hyperpathia' or 'dysaesthesiae'. The abnormal, heightened sensitivity can make the life of the patient very miserable; this complication is

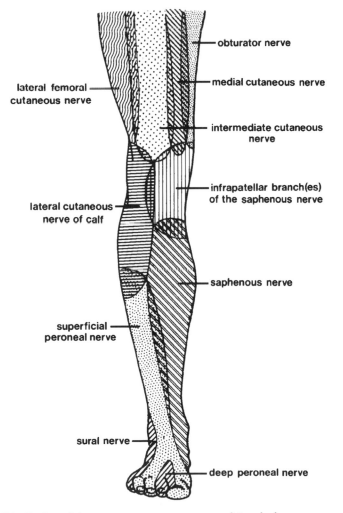

Figure 2.5 Distribution of the sensory cutaneous nerves supplying the leg

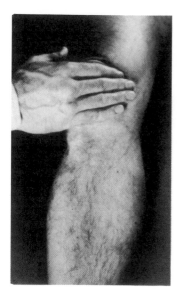

Figure 2.6 Small amounts of synovial fluid can be swept up into the suprapatellar pouch by the flat of the hand; the return of fluid into the medial hollow can usually be discerned

particularly troublesome in younger women, and it may prove very difficult to correct surgically. If a neuroma of the nerve appears to be present, defined by its location to one side along the line of the nerve, and the exquisite tenderness and radiation of sensation in the distribution of the nerve provoked by tapping it with the finger (Tinel sign), then there may be an indication to explore the nerve. However, the outcome of such surgery is never predictable, even if every effort is taken to bury the proximal stump of the damaged nerve securely into adjacent tibial bone.

Effusion

Major effusion   Gradation of the volumes of an effusion is possible if a major effusion is taken to be present when the fluid can easily be identified distending the suprapatellar pouch with the knees straight (Figure 2.6).

It is quite unnecessary in this case to attempt to produce a 'patellar tap', although it will be present. The patellar tap test is so often misinterpreted or is falsely positive that it is better ignored. Using the medial hollow of the knee, evident in most people at the level of the patella, the presence or absence of a fluid shift at this site can now be checked (Plates 1 and 2). A major effusion will of course fill this space completely so that no hollowing is present.

Moderate effusion   A moderate effusion will fill the medial hollow of its own accord after the examining hand has swept fluid upwards into the patellar pouch (Figure 2.6). The fluid shift or thrill should readily be seen by viewing the medial side of the joint tangentially in good light.

Minor effusion   In a minor effusion the trace of fluid present will not fill the hollow visibly unless, after sweeping fluid upwards, the examiner then empties the suprapatellar pouch actively. This shift of fluid is best achieved by compressing the lateral gutter and then the lateral side of the suprapatellar pouch with the back of the hand, again using a sweeping motion.

The hand should not be taken too far medially over the suprapatellar pouch as it may then obscure the medial hollow. With experience, each examiner develops his own technique for eliciting fluid and no single method is best for demonstrating this sign. It may help to flex and extend the knee a few times, thereby pumping fluid forwards from the posterior recesses of the joint, before palpating for fluid.

Patellofemoral joint

The final assessment with the knee extended concerns the patellofemoral joint. When the patient relaxes completely, the quadriceps muscle will no longer tether the patella within its groove. Since the knee cap can then be moved from side to side, this permits the examining fingers to palpate up to one-half of the posterior surface, partly medially and partly laterally. Tenderness may be remarked upon by the patient, and apprehension is shown both to this manoeuvre and also on deviating the patella laterally, forcing it passively against the lateral femoral condyle.

Patellar apprehension   The 'patellar apprehension test' may be so strongly positive that the patient withdraws the leg rapidly as the examiner

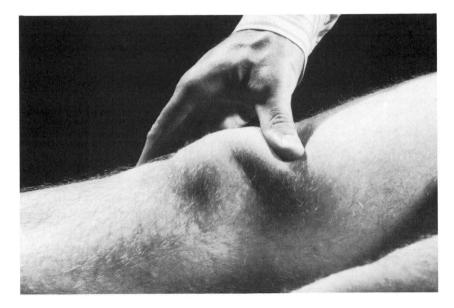

Figure 2.7 the patellar restraint test

approaches the knee with his hand, thus preventing any contact. The interpretation of such a florid reaction is difficult, and although it may mean that a subluxing patella is the source of the symptoms, the patient may also be responding in an inappropriate way emotionally; the surgeon should then be wary about recommending a surgical solution too readily.

Patellar grind and patellar restraint tests If the patient permits the patella to be palpated, discomfort can be assessed by compressing or grinding the posterior patellar surface against the femoral condyles, comparing the test to the opposite knee.

A more vigorous test of retropatellar pain is afforded by the 'patellar restraint' test. The patella, still with the leg extended, is trapped in the femoral groove with the thumb or hand of the examiner. While the superior patellar pole is pushed distally the patient is asked to straighten the knee (Figure 2.7). Since the patella is not free to move upwards in the femoral groove, a resultant force is generated backwards, thus compressing the patella forcibly against the femur.

Acute pain is felt if a patellar syndrome is present, but the opposite side should always be tested since bilateral pain is often elicited. It is rarely as acute on the asymptomatic side; however, the fact that this sign is positive in both knees is an expression of the fact that patellar dysfunction is usually bilateral to some degree.

Movement (tracking and crepitus) The hand should now be placed, palm downwards, upon the knee cap and the joint flexed and extended. Crepitus may be both felt and heard, but is so regularly evident in asymptomatic knees that this feature is not of diagnostic value on its own. Indeed, many patients with marked patellofemoral crepitus present with completely normal contiguous articular cartilage surfaces when reviewed through the arthroscope.

An assessment of patellar tracking should be made at this stage; a degree of side-to-side movement or a frank lateral subluxation of the patella may be seen in both extension and flexion.

Flexed knee

The knee is now flexed to a right angle. This throws into relief the contours of the femur and tibia, and the joint lines and points of ligament attachment can be palpated precisely. A knowledge of the surface anatomy of the knee is essential (see Figures 1.2 and 1.3) and if care is taken with this part of the examination much useful detail can be elicited.

Joint lines

The joint lines lie at 90° to the shin and are level with the lower pole of the patella. If the knee is plump it is difficult to see the small indentation produced by the hollow of the articular margins, but surface landmarks and firm palpation should make the joint line apparent. Since this line represents the peripheral margin of the meniscus and its anchoring meniscotibial ligament, it is of paramount importance to identify this region. Careful, fingertip pressure over discrete portions of both the lateral and medial joint lines yields a great deal of information about both the condition of the menisci and the possibility of an arthritic process (see Plate 6).

Ligaments

There is a 'no man's land' medially where the medial collateral ligament crosses the joint line. Tenderness here, or posterolaterally, may arise from the relevant ligament, from the meniscus, or from both structures. Palpation along the line of the ligaments will help to determine whether a tear of the ligament is likely. Therefore, feel the adductor tubercle proximally and the tibial flare distally, in order to identify the point of maximum sensitivity. Laterally, the fibular collateral ligament is more posteriorly placed, running from the lateral femoral condyle to the fibular head (see Plate 7). Injury to the iliotibial tract may cause a similar, superimposed tender spot, but this is relatively rare. Capsular tenderness may be widespread or localized, and the margins of patella, femur and tibia should be palpated thoroughly for the possibility of symptomatic synovial fringe lesions, caused by entrapment of the synovium. The fat-pad may occasionally be tender, and thickenings of the synovial shelves may be present (see Figure 2.8), with a clicking sensation over the medial femoral condyle during knee flexion if the shelf, or plica, has enlarged because of chronic irritation and fibrosis.

The largest of these plicae runs medial and roughly parallel to the patella, from the upper pole of the patella to the fat-pad. Within the suprapatellar pouch are the medial and lateral suprapatellar plicae, which represent the residual portions of a diaphragm of synovium which separated the pouch from the rest of the cavity of the knee in embryonic life. The ligamentum

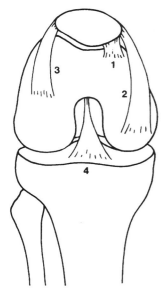

Figure 2.8 *Sites of the synovial folds or plicae: 1 – medial suprapatellar plica; 2 – medial synovial shelf; 3 – lateral synovial shelf; 4 – ligamentum mucosum (alar ligament). Other synovial fibrous bands may form as a result of direct trauma*

mucosum, or alar ligament, is also a synovial fold or prolongation normally found in the knee. These structures are only pathological when they become sufficiently thickened to rub against the condyles.

Bone

Palpation of the femoral and tibial condyles sometimes elicits acute tenderness, and the differential diagnosis in these instances includes osteomyelitis, osteochondritis dissecans, bone or cartilage tumours (see Chapter 9) and a fracture (see Chapter 8). The presence of tenderness which spreads into the femoral and tibial shafts should alert one to the possibility of a more extensive lesion, although after injury the patient may find it difficult to localize tenderness precisely. In some apprehensive individuals, tenderness may be commented upon virtually anywhere one cares to palpate, and obviously this hypersensitive response must be recognized and placed in perspective.

MOVEMENT

The final stage in examining the knee when the patient is on a couch or bench consists of moving the joint, not only to see if the normal range is present, but to assess whether there is any abnormal motion or laxity. The ranges of movement of the knee should be recalled and passively tested in turn:

- Extension to flexion (an arc of approximately 150°)
- Rotation (approximately 20°)
- Coronal movement into valgus and varus (a few degrees each way)
- Sagittal motion (rarely more than 2 or 3 millimetres)

Of course, these movements vary between people and hence the opposite knee should be used as the reference measurement.

Extension

The degree of extension, or hyperextension, is accurately measured with the patient lying prone. This test ensures that even a few degrees of loss of movement are noted, and also affords an opportunity to view the back of the knee (see Plate 8). The patient is asked to hang the legs straight out, with the front of the knees at the edge of the examining couch. It is essential that this edge is firm and that the legs are placed symmetrically, so that the comparison between the injured and normal knees is fair. Any slight elevation of the heel on the affected side indicates a loss of full extension, and the eye is far better equipped to assess a distance of this sort than in attempting to detect a minor alteration in angle. A number of small but significant losses of extension, in many cases representing a locked knee, will be missed if the legs are examined with the patient only supine, and on a soft bed.

Increased extension, or hyperextension, is encountered in the individual with ligament laxity. If the increase is present unilaterally it may represent a tear of one or both cruciate ligaments, or laxity of the posterior capsule, secondary to trauma.

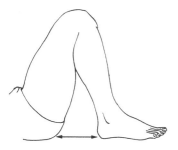

Figure 2.9 Minor losses of knee flexion are best measured by the heel to buttock distance, comparing each leg in turn. Greater restriction of flexion should be measured with a goniometer

Flexion

Flexion is measured with the patient supine or prone, using the heel-to-buttock distance on each side, measured in finger-breadths, rather than attempting to estimate an angle (see Plate 9). Viewed from the side of the patient these differences may be compared to the opposite leg, since small but measurable losses of flexion are of great significance when formulating a diagnosis (see Figure 2.9).

Greater restrictions of flexion, when the knee can flex little more than to a right angle, are better measured with a clinical goniometer. This simple instrument is very useful when monitoring recovery of knee movement after injury. However, it is not always available, and hence a careful comparison with the opposite leg is still an effective yet easy method of examining the flexion arc.

Collateral ligament laxity

Knee in slight flexion

Coronal laxity implicates the collateral ligaments and capsule. However, if this form of laxity is excessive other ligamentous structures are usually also injured. Valgus and varus stress should be applied at first with the knee in 20° of flexion (see Plate 11–13). This relaxes the posterior capsule and means that stability is principally reliant upon the medial or lateral structures. Rupture of the lateral restraints – the lateral collateral ligament, the fascia lata, the biceps femoris and popliteus muscles, and the arcuate complex – results in moderate varus laxity; this increases perceptibly when the cruciate ligaments are stretched or torn.

It is difficult to grade laxity precisely, and the knee tends to rotate and flex during the attempt at assessment, thus complicating the measurement. However, the following grades are generally accepted:

- Grade I (minor) – the joint tilts by up to 5 mm more than the contralateral side, with a slight suction sign (a 'jog' of movement)
- Grade II (moderate) – abnormal movement of between 5 and 10 mm is possible, and the suction sign is marked (laxity with 'end point')
- Grade III (severe) – more than 10 mm of opening up is possible, sometimes with no feeling of an 'end point' since tissue resistance is minimal (laxity with no 'end point')

Examination under a general anaesthetic is recommended if there is doubt about the extent of the abnormal laxity.

Knee in extension

When the knee is extended the medial side will only hinge open if there is a torn cruciate ligament in addition to the injured medial collateral ligament and the medial capsule. Usually it is the anterior cruciate ligament which is ruptured, and if the posterior cruciate is progressively torn the valgus laxity will increase. Although the brunt of an injury may be borne by one structure, causing macroscopic tearing, other soft tissues of the knee are invariably stretched and partially ruptured. Thus, tears of the medial ligament are

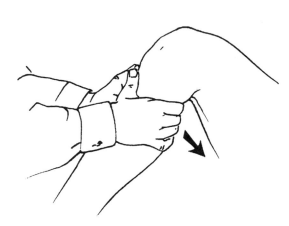

Figure 2.10 *Stretching of the posterior cruciate ligament allows the tibia to sublux posteriorly ('drop-back')*

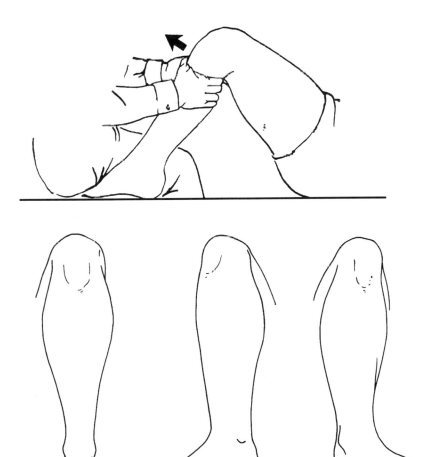

Figure 2.11 *Anterior drawer tests with modifications to show rotatory laxity [1, tibia in a neutral position; 2, tibia in external rotation (assessing anteromedial laxity); 3, tibia in internal rotation (assessing anterolateral laxity)]*

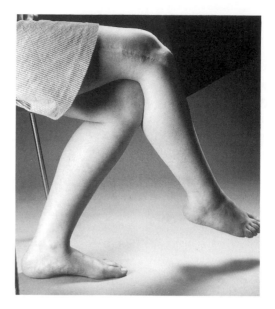

Figure 2.12 The 'crossed knee test' allows the hamstrings to relax naturally, demonstrating anterior laxity

often accompanied by synovial disruption, rents in the posteromedial capsule, and by damage to the anterior cruciate ligament and medial meniscus.

Since ligaments are not simply passive restrainers of abnormal movement, but also carry nerve fibres concerned with proprioception and pain, complete tears may render the knee relatively painless when it is manipulated. In these cases, the synovial envelope is usually incompetent and there is a characteristic lack of a tense haemarthrosis. Instead, a boggy swelling overlies the site of rupture, and an ecchymosis develops rapidly and spreads widely (see Figure 2.2). The loss of these normal controls means that the knee wobbles during passive flexion and extension, and rotatory motion to an abnormal degree is evident. The full complexity of these pathological changes are only now beginning to be elucidated, and are discussed further in Chapter 5.

Cruciate ligament laxity

Laxity in the sagittal plane has been taught classically as a differentiation between the anterior and posterior drawer tests. These two assessments are carried out with the knee in 90° of flexion and, prior to any attempt at producing abnormal movement, the anterior contour of the knee should be viewed from the lateral side (Figure 2.10). If there is tibial 'dropback' a concavity is seen below the patella where the tibia has sagged back posteriorly. This indicates that the posterior cruciate ligament has been torn or elongated after a partial rupture, such as is produced when the proximal tibia is thrust forcibly backwards in a collision or from hyperextension of the knee. This sign may be wrongly construed as a positive anterior drawer sign, since the tibia can be drawn forwards to its rightful position.

After assessing the lateral tibiofemoral relationship, the hamstrings should be palpated to ensure that they are relaxed and then the tibia firmly moved anteriorly and posteriorly by grasping it with both hands just below the joint line (Figures 2.11 and 2.12; see also Plates 18 and 19). The foot should be secured by the examiner who either sits upon the side of it or applies his elbow against the dorsum of the foot. Increased movement of more than a few millimetres anteriorly or posteriorly, compared to the other knee, indicates that abnormal laxity is present. Unfortunately, a positive anterior drawer sign rarely results from an anterior cruciate ligament tear alone, and usually there is laxity of the posteromedial corner of the knee. A more specific test of anterior cruciate deficiency is the 'Lachman' test, which should be combined with dynamic assessment of tibiofemoral subluxation under load.

Ritchey–Lachman test

The Ritchey–Lachman test allows the examiner to assess anterior laxity accurately, comparing it to the contralateral knee. In 20–30° of flexion the restraint afforded by the posterior meniscal horns and the collateral structures is reduced, in comparison to the 90° drawer test. Torg *et al.* (1976) popularized the test which was recognized as early as 1875 by Georges Noulis (Pässler, 1993) and reported by Ritchey (1960) as a useful means of assessing anterior cruciate ligament disruption.

The anterior stress is applied manually (see Plate 20) or with a standardized 89 N force. Normally there should be no more than 3 mm variation between the knees, and less than this distance is difficult to perceive on standard, clinical examination. Four grades of increasing laxity are recognized (Gurtler *et al.*, 1987):

- Grade I (3–6 mm) – palpable subluxation with a soft end point
- Grade II (6–9 mm) – visible subluxation with a soft end point
- Grade III (9–16 mm) – passive subluxation when the proximal tibial is supported
- Grade IV (16 20 mm) – active subluxation produced by quadriceps and gastrocnemius contraction

The test is usually performed with the patient supine, and the examiner uses both hands. This may prove difficult if the leg is large and muscular or if the examiner has small hands. Modifications have therefore been proposed, including the supported test (see Plate 14) (Strobel and Stedtfeld, 1990) and testing the patient lying on the uninjured side, which may also allow the patient to show active (grade IV) subluxation more readily (see Plate 15). If the laxity is gross, the crossed knee test is often positive (Figure 2.12) and has the advantage that both knees can be compared under similar load, namely the weight of the leg, and the patient is willing to relax fully in a familiar sitting posture.

The prone Lachman test (Feagin, 1988) and the Hackenbruch modification (Hackenbruch and Müller, 1987) rely upon the thigh being stabilized while the tibia is manipulated with one or both hands, respectively. The test can be carried out at the time of the prone-lying assessment of joint extension. Finochietto (1935) recognized a snapping or jerking sensation caused by a torn or hypermobile posterior meniscal horn as an additional characteristic of the pathological anterior tibial glide and this

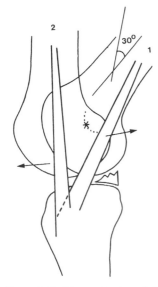

Figure 2.13 The mechanism of the anterior pivot (jerk) test relies upon the forward subluxation of the lateral tibial plateau under the convexity of the femoral condyle

sensation can sometimes be reinforced by rotating the tibia internally or externally, either with the patient prone or supine. The joint lines should be palpated concurrently.

The pivot shift (jerk) test

This test is pathognomonic of symptomatic anterolateral laxity, for the sense of lateral tibial condylar subluxation is disabling. The knee buckles or gives way, with the sensation of the knuckles of one hand moving forcibly over the knuckles of the opposite hand. The instability was recognized by Amédée Bonnet in 1845 (Pässler, 1993) and later by Hey-Groves (1919). Lemaire (1967) demonstrated the subluxation of the knee but it only became extensively recognized in English publications after the paper by Galway *et al.* (1972). A number of variations have been described and may prove bewildering.

- Slocum test (Slocum *et al.*, 1976)
  (a) patient lies on the normal side with that hip and knee flexed (1976)
  (b) the knee to be examined is extended fully with the medial side of the foot resting on the couch
  (c) a valgus force is applied to the knee with the tibia internally rotated
  (d) as the knee is flexed actively to 30°, the anterior subluxation of the lateral tibial condyle is reduced
- McIntosh test (Galway *et al.*, 1972)
  (a) patient lies supine
  (b) the knee is extended by supporting the leg with a hand under the heel
  (c) the lateral tibial condyle subluxes anteriorly, and this is made more obvious by applying a valgus force to the knee with the other hand
  (d) passive flexion of the knee will reduce the subluxation
- Losee test (Losee, 1983)
  (a) patient lies supine
  (b) with the knee flexed 50–60° a valgus force is applied
  (c) the knee is slowly extended and pressure is also applied behind the head of the fibula
  (d) a clunk occurs as the lateral tibia subluxes forwards during the last few degrees towards full extension
- Noyes test (Noyes and Groody, 1988) ('flexion–rotation drawer test')
  (a) patient lies supine
  (b) examiner supports the extended leg at the calf, allowing the femur to rotate externally and drop posteriorly if laxity is present
  (c) the anterior subluxation of the lateral tibial plateau relative to the femur is corrected by gently flexing the knee while pushing the upper shin posteriorly
  (d) a clunk may be felt

These tests produce a jerk or 'pivot shift' as the lateral tibial condyle alters its arc of movement in relation to the femur (Figures 2.13 and 2.14). The essential components of any of these tests are:

- A relaxed patient (hamstring spasm will prevent the subluxation)
- Sufficient laxity to allow the lateral tibial condyle to alter its relationship to the femur during the last 30° of knee movement towards extension
- An additional valgus stress to make the subluxation more obvious. The application of an axial force to the foot, directed upwards, mimics weightbearing and will accentuate the abnormal subluxation (Figures 2.15 and 2.16). The convex surface of the lateral tibial condyle promotes the sudden nature of the subluxation or jerk (see Plates 21–23).

It is important to become familiar with one form of the test and to practise it regularly. The flexion–rotation drawer test may allow better assessment of the jerk in the acutely injured knee and the essential feature of the examination is that protective hamstring spasm or tone should be minimized. In order to emphasize the subluxation, valgus stress and axially loading are required, together with internal rotation of the tibia. Rupture of the iliotibial tract, obstruction from a meniscal tear or degenerative changes prevent the pivot shift, and it may be seen normally in some children, particularly in the presence of a discoid lateral meniscus, and in adults with ligament hyperlaxity.

In assessing the pivot shift test, conventional grading describes a negative test (grade 0), a pivot slide (grade I) where the tibial subluxation is checked before it extends beyond the zenith of the lateral tibial condyle, and a

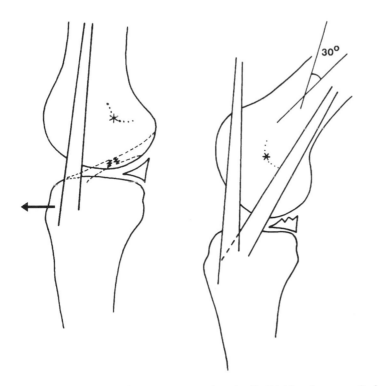

Figure 2.14 The pivot shift or jerk test is positive when the iliotibial band comes to lie behind the pivot of the femur while the knee is flexed from 0° to 30°, thus producing a palpable (and usually visible) reduction of the anteriorly subluxed lateral tibial condyle. This forward and backward motion eventually damages the secondary restraints.

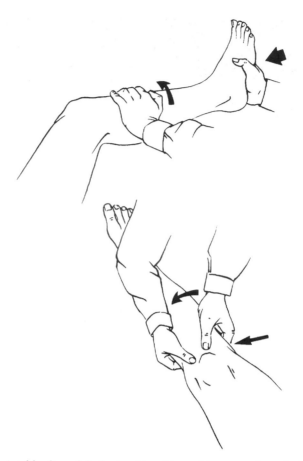

Figure 2.15 *Axial loading of the leg is achieved by pushing upwards on the foot, or by applying pressure through the knee to the stabilized hip*

complete shift or jerk (grade II). The grade III pivot is gross, with 'hang up' during reduction and significant discomfort. Jakob *et al.* (1987) graded the test in relation to the position of the tibia, and suggest that this helps to demonstrate disruption of the posteromedial and posterolateral structures (grade III). Their grade I pivot shift is a palpable rather than visible tibial subluxation, present only when the tibia is internally rotated. Grade II subluxation is evident with the tibia in internal or neutral rotation, but absent with external tibial rotation. The grade III test is markedly positive even with the tibia externally rotated and indicates a significant degree of laxity of the secondary restraints.

Control of the pivot shift, either by improved hamstring tone or by anterior cruciate ligament reconstruction, correlates closely with successful elimination of instability. Increasing medial laxity and complex instability patterns make it increasingly difficult to prevent the pivot phenomenon, but it is essential that the patient learns to avoid the episodes of subluxation. Proprioceptive education (Barrett, 1991) and altered gait patterns will help, but in many cases a change in sporting activity is the only remedy. When

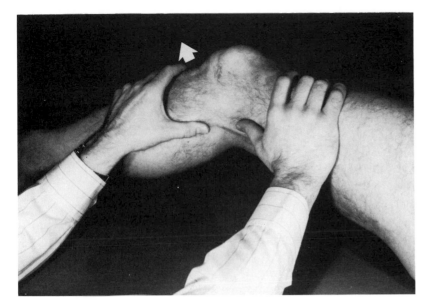

Figure 2.16(a) *Anterior subluxation of the lateral tibial condyle can be produced by pressure behind the head of the fibula*

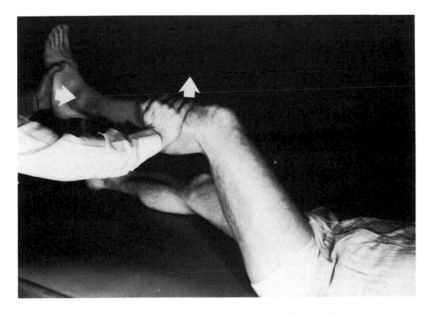

Figure 2.16(b) *The 'jerk' or 'pivot shift' test (see Table 4.3 and Figs. 4.10 and 4.11).*

giving way occurs regularly in everyday tasks, and meniscal and chondral lesions develop secondarily, it is hard to avoid the conclusion that only surgical reconstruction will suffice.

The genu recurvatum–external rotation test (see Figure 5.13) assesses the integrity of the posterolateral structures. The definition of the pathology is complex and a dynamic portrayal of the laxity may be revealed by the reverse pivot shift test. This can be carried out with the patient supine, prone or lying on the uninjured side, but grading is more difficult than with the anterior pivot shift or jerk.

Tests of meniscal integrity

A torn meniscus produces joint line tenderness, often very localized, an effusion, which may be localized, as well as the more common total intrasynovial swelling, and locking. The last term describes not simply a loss of full extension, but also restriction of flexion and rotation. The loss of extension is rarely more than 10–20°, and a greater loss suggests some other pathological lesion. In approximately 70% of cases these are the three cardinal signs of a torn meniscus.

Joint line fullness or the presence of a discrete swelling indicates meniscal pathology, often in association with localized synovitis. A lateral meniscal cyst is much more common than a medial cyst, although a pedunculated tag of medial meniscus may sometimes lodge in the medial gutter, above or below the meniscotibial ligament, producing a variable, firm swelling in the vicinity of the medial joint line. The snapping knee produced by a discoid lateral meniscus (see page 108) is also a characteristic finding.

Stress can be applied to the meniscus by Bragard's sign, in which medial meniscal tenderness is accentuated by externally rotating and extending the tibia, at the same time as compressing the anterior horn with a finger. Valgus or varus stress may also produce meniscal tenderness on the side of the concavity (Bohler's sign), although this test is ambiguous. When combined with altering flexion of the knee (the 'D' test) a more accurate meniscal assessment is possible.

Finochietto's 'jump sign' (Finochietto, 1935) is positive in the lax knee when anteroposterior drawer movement causes a snap or jerk.

The McMurray test   The McMurray test (McMurray, 1928) for a torn meniscus has a time-honoured place in the examination of the knee. The examiner should palpate the joint line with the fingers of one hand (Figure 2.17) while at the same time the tibia is rotated beneath the femur. The heel of the foot can be gripped conveniently and this allows both internal rotation and external rotation of the tibia, with the knee placed in successively increasing degrees of flexion.

A positive test is present when a clunk can be felt. The production of pain is not in itself diagnostic as this can occur with ligament injury, unaccompanied by any meniscal pathology. When truly positive, the test is of diagnostic value and the patient will often remark that a feeling of locking has been produced. Indeed, forcible manipulation of the knee may precipitate locking in a knee where an intermittent history of meniscal displacement has been obtained.

A negative McMurray test does not rule out meniscal pathology, since the manoeuvre depends upon the displacement of an unstable meniscal segment, and also upon the experience of the examiner and the ability of the patient to relax. Posterior third vertical tears of the meniscus are classically those that produce a clunking sensation, which can be both palpated and often heard during the McMurray test. With the advent of the arthroscope, the test is of less value. The Apley test, (Apley and Solomon, 1994), whereby an attempt is made to distinguish between a ligamentous injury (by distracting the knee) and a meniscal injury (by axial compression of the knee), is open to considerable misinterpretation and is not recommended for the assessment of an acute soft-tissue injury of the knee.

The bounce test (see Plate 10) assesses the feel of the knee as it is dropped into full extension. Loss of the normal screw-home action of the femur upon the tibia may be detected as a painful 'bounce' of the knee out of its fully extended position. Passive loss of flexion, measured by the heel-to-buttock distance (see Plate 9), and extension, measured by the prone-lying test (see Plate 8), are important discriminators between the presence or absence of

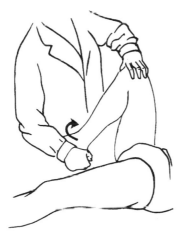

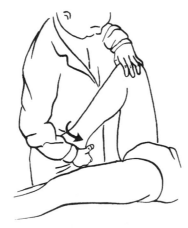

Figure 2.17 The McMurray test for an obstructing posterior meniscal tear. The joint line should be palpated for a clunk, while the tibia is rotated with the knee in different degrees of flexion

obstructive pathology, although effusions, synovitis, arthritis, loose bodies and protective muscle spasm may produce similar losses of movement. Voluntary restriction of extension and flexion, however, tend to be more gross than the subtle losses of movement caused by chronic meniscal lesions.

These tests for meniscal pathology are open to misinterpretation but are sometimes confirmatory. Eliciting pain by these manoeuvres is not pathognomic of a meniscal tear, but the production of a clunk or abnormal movement may cause the patient to remark that the symptoms of instability have been reproduced. It is always as well to check that a similar clunk cannot be elicited in the opposite knee, and examination of the knee on different occasions is recommended, particularly if the assessments are separated by a few weeks. There is certainly nothing to suggest that such delay will adversely influence the eventual outcome.

Weightbearing tests   A full squat is impossible when an obstructive or painful meniscal tear is present (see Plate 16). The distance between the heel and the buttock during squatting should be carefully checked in comparison with the normal side. A 'duck waddle' adds further stress to the abnormal knee and is a useful discriminant between the knee that is seriously compromised and one that may not require arthroscopic intervention. This test can also be performed with the knee partially flexed; the patient is asked to rotate internally and externally on the loaded knee (see Plate 17). Apprehension, pain, local tenderness and the presence of a clunk are noted.

CONCLUSION

In conclusion, examination of the knee should include inspection, careful palpation of all anatomical landmarks, and a description of the passive and active ranges of movement in the knee. Flexion and extension are best measured by means of the heel-to-buttock distance and the prone-lying test, respectively, and a comparison between the range of rotation, forward and backward glide, and coronal movement should be carefully made with the opposite knee as the normal baseline. In the early stages after injury, both meniscal and ligament damage may restrict movement, and the separation of these two interlinked pathologies is often difficult and sometimes unnecessary. In the later stages of convalescence, unstable meniscal tears generally produce losses of movement in all planes, whereas ligamentous laxity will result in pathologically increased ranges of movement.

References

Apley, A.G. and Solomon, L. (1994) *A System of Orthopaedics and Fractures*, 7th edn, Oxford, Butterworth-Heinemann

Barrett, D.S. (1991) Proprioception and function after anterior cruciate reconstruction. *J. Bone Joint Surg.*,**73B**, 833–887

Feagin, J.A. (1988) Principles of diagnosis and treatment. In *The Crucial Ligaments. Diagnosis and Treatment of Ligamentous Injuries About the Knee* (ed. Feagin, J.A.) Churchill Livingstone, New York, pp. 261–285

Finochietto, R. (1935) Semilunar cartilages of the knee. The 'Jump Sign'. *J. Bone Joint Surg.*, **17A**, 916–918

Galway, R., Beaupre, A. and McIntosh, D.L. (1972) Pivot-shift – a clinical sign of symptomatic anterior cruciate insufficiency. *J. Bone Joint Surg.*, **54B**, 763–764

Gurtler, R.A., Stine, R. and Torg, J.S. (1987) Lachman test evaluated – quantification of a clinical observation. *Clin Orthop*. **216**, 141–150

Hackenbruch, W. and Müller, W. (1987) Untersuchung des Kniegelenkes. *Orthopäde*, **16**, 100–112

Hey-Groves, E. (1919) The crucial ligaments of the knee joint; their function, rupture and the operative treatment of the same. *Br. J. Surg*, **7**, 505–515

Jakob, R.P., Stäubli, H.U. and Deland, J.T. (1987) Grading the pivot shift. *J. Bone Joint Surg.*, **69B**, 294–299

Lemaire, M. (1967) Ruptures anciennes du ligament croisé antérior du genou. *J. Chir.* (Paris), **93**, 311–320

Losee, R.E. (1983) Concepts of the pivot-shift. *Clin. Orthop*, **172**, 45–51

McMurray, T.P. (1928) The diagnosis of internal derangements of the knee. In: *Robert Jones Birthday Volume*, Oxford Medical Publications, Oxford, pp. 301–305

Noyes, F.R. and Grood, E.S. (1988) Diagnosis of knee ligament injuries: clinical concepts. In: *The Crucial Ligaments. Diagnosis and Treatment of Ligamentous Injuries About the Knee* (ed. Feagin, J.A.) Churchill Livingstone, New York, pp. 261–285

Pässler, H.H. (1993) The history of the cruciate ligaments : some forgotten (or unknown) facts from Europe. *Knee Surg. Sports Traumatol. Arthroscopy*, **1**, 13–16

Ritchey, S.J. (1960) Ligamentous disruption of the knee. A review with analysis of 28 cases. *US Armed Forces Med. J.*, **11**, 167–176

Slocum, D.B., James, S.l., Larson, R.L. and Singer, K.M. (1976) Clinical test for anterolateral instability of the knee. *Clin. Orthop.*, **118**, 63–69

Strobel, M. and Stedtfeld, H.W. (1990) *Diagnostic Evaluation of the Knee*, Springer-Verlag, Berlin, p. 121

Torg, J.S., Conrad, W. and Kalen, V. (1976) Clinical diagnosis of anterior cruciate ligament instability in the athlete. *Am. J. Sports Med.*, **4**, 84–91

3

Investigations

BLOOD TESTS – SYNOVIAL FLUID ANALYSIS – BIOPSY –
RADIOGRAPHY – ARTHROGRAPHY – ARTHROSCOPY –
RADIOISOTOPE IMAGING – COMPUTERIZED TOMOGRAPHY
– VENOGRAPHY AND ARTERIOGRAPHY – MAGNETIC
RESONANCE – CYBEX DYNAMOMETRY – EXERCISE TESTS

BLOOD TESTS

The investigation of a patient with a painful knee, particularly if swelling
and stiffness are present, should attempt to exclude systemic disease. When
an inflammatory arthritis is suspected, the full blood count, erythrocyte
sedimentation rate, C-reactive protein, rheumatoid and antinuclear factors,
and titres against various antigens should be obtained. Metabolic abnormalities may also produce an arthropathy and therefore electrolytes, blood
glucose and uric acid levels should be assessed. If a blood dyscrasia is
suspected, tests for clotting, including factors VIII and IX, and for sickle
cell anaemia should be conducted. Occasionally, venereal arthropathy may
produce symptoms in a joint, and serological tests to exclude gonococcal
and syphilitic infections should be carried out. The medical implications of
these conditions are discussed further in Chapter 9.

SYNOVIAL FLUID ANALYSIS

Synovial fluid can be analysed after aspirating a few millimetres from the
knee. The pH of fluid, together with its contents of lactate, fat or blood are
important in the differential diagnosis (Table 3.1). The presence of crystals
should be sought if a uric acid or pyrophosphate arthropathy is suspected.

The white cell count in the synovial fluid is of some differential diagnostic value in that osteoarthritis produces a monocytic picture, with less than
2×10^9 cells per litre and relatively normal complement levels. Rheumatoid
arthritis results in a predominance of polymorphonuclear white cells, with
a count of $4–50 \times 10^9$ cells per litre, and low levels of complement. In septic
arthritis the polymorphonuclear cell count is very much higher, usually
exceeding 60×10^9 cells per litre. An inflammatory condition also lowers
the viscosity of the synovial fluid and increases the total protein content,
such that there is a tendency to form a spontaneous clot.

Table 3.1 Synovial fluid analysis as an aid to diagnosis

Blood	Fracture, ligament rupture, synovial tear (haemophilia, haemangioma)
Fat	Osteochondral fracture, fat-pad lesion
Debris	Articular cartilage damage including chondromalacia, meniscal tear
Cells	(a) Monocyte predominance in osteoarthritis
	(b) Polymorphonuclear cell predominance in inflammatory synovitis including rheumatoid arthritis and septic arthritis
Crystals	(a) Gout (urate) – feathery crystals
	(b) Pseudogout (monophosphate) – rectangular crystals
Lactate, acidity and lysosomal enzymes	Increased in inflammatory conditions
Complement	(a) Increased in Reiter's syndrome and gout
	(b) Increased in osteoarthritis
	(c) Decreased in rheumatoid arthritis

Synovial fluid should be subjected to microscopy, employing both the standard Gram stain and Ziehl–Nielsen staining for acid–alcohol fast bacilli. When infection is suspected, the microscopic appearances may be of great value in early diagnosis, with later confirmation of the bacterial cause of the infection by means of culture. Both pyogenic and tuberculous organisms should be suspected, with the use of appropriate culture media.

BIOPSY

The arthroscope has made 'closed' synovial and articular cartilage biopsy relatively simple (see Chapter 9). Bone biopsy is only possible by means of an operation under general anaesthesia, and with a tourniquet in place. Bone should be obtained both from the lesion and from the contiguous border of the normal bone after appropriate preoperative investigations and imaging.

RADIOGRAPHY

Radiographs of the knee complement the history and clinical examination, and are an essential part of any assessment, despite Smillie's contention: 'It should be stated, and repeated, that there is no human joint less related, in terms of function, to radiographic findings than the knee joint' (Smillie, 1980). After any significant injury which produces persisting symptoms, a radiograph is advisable, and should also precede investigations such as arthroscopy. A standard anteroposterior view (Figure 3.1) is often augmented by a standing film, showing femorotibial alignment during weightbearing.

A lateral film is taken with the knee in 30° of flexion (Figure 3.2; see also Figure 7.6), although a view of the knee fully extended is of value

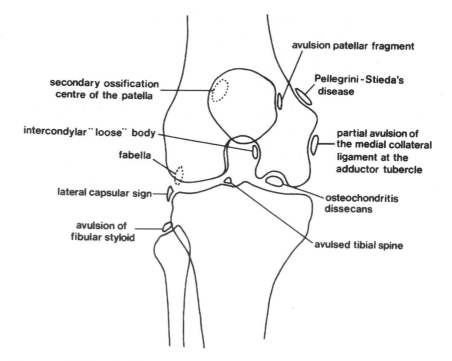

Figure 3.1 Radiographic lesions apparent on an anteroposterior radiograph

when the position of the patella is being assessed in relation to the femoral condyles. A lipohaemarthrosis can be demonstrated using a horizontal beam when the patient is lying supine, the fat layer separating from the more dense blood. Radiographs may also be used to assess the 'resting position of the knee' and to assess the degree of flexion contracture or flexion limitation.

The signs of an effusion include:

- An anterior shift or tilting of the patella
- Widening of the suprapatellar pouch
- Anterior bulging of the patellar ligament
- Distension of the posterior capsule

However, the volume of fluid required to produce these signs is usually quite gross and clinical assessment remains the best method of defining the volume of fluid within the knee.

Skyline view

The axial, tangential or 'skyline' patellar view shows the retropatellar space and the relationship between the patella and the femoral condyles at one particular level (Table 3.2). Too much can be made of the patellar characteristics and the congruency of the patellofemoral joint since these are known to vary according to the amount of knee flexion. A variety of patellar outlines has been described (Figure 3.4) but these are a poor indicator of true patellar shape and the dynamics of the patellofemoral joint. The

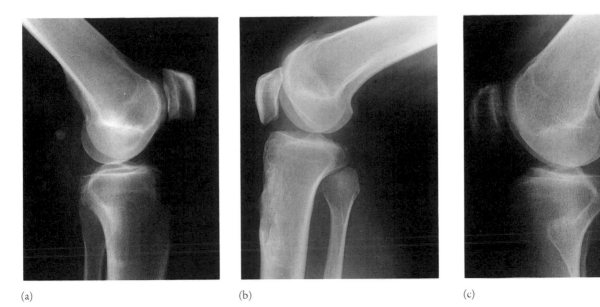

(a)   (b)   (c)

Figure 3.2 A popliteal cyst is outlined by radio opaque bodies (a), patella baja (b) and a plasmacytoma of the patella (c)

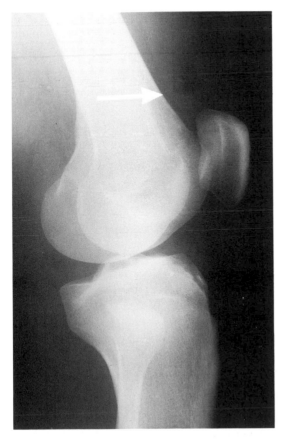

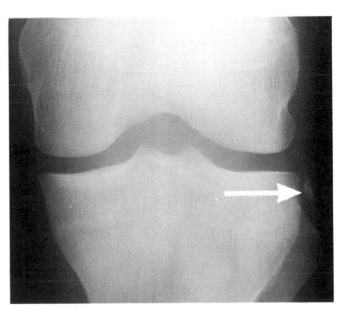

Figure 3.3(a) A haemarthrosis is evident from the fluid level that has formed in the suprapatellar pouch

Figure 3.3(b) The Segond fracture (lateral capsular avulsion) seen after anterior cruciate ligament injury

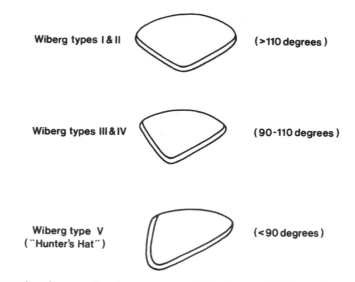

Wiberg types I & II   (>110 degrees)

Wiberg types III & IV   (90–110 degrees)

Wiberg type V
("Hunter's Hat")   (<90 degrees)

Figure 3.4 *Three basic patellar shapes are recognizable, but are of dubious relevance to clinical conditions*

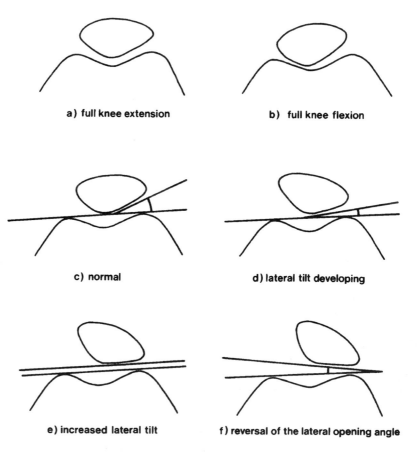

a) full knee extension   b) full knee flexion

c) normal   d) lateral tilt developing

e) increased lateral tilt   f) reversal of the lateral opening angle

Figure 3.5 *Different facets of the patella articulate with the femoral condyles during knee flexion (a,b). Increasing lateral patellar tilt may be associated with lateral subluxation (c–f) and is measured by the lateral opening angle on a skyline view with the knee in 30–40° of flexion*

Table 3.2 Tangential ('skyline') radiographic views of the patellofemoral joint

1	Knee fully flexed ('sunrise view')	Shows 'odd facet' of patella articulating with medial femoral condylar groove
2	Knee flexed 45° (Hughston view) (tube angle of 30°)	Shows patellofemoral articulation and intercondylar notch, but some distortion occurs due to the angulation
3	Knee flexed to 30° (Merchant view) (radiographic plate on shin)	Useful demonstration of the intercondylar notch and congruence angle
4	Knee flexed 30° (Laurin view) (radiographic plate on anterior thigh)	Easier to obtain than the Merchant view, and as useful but the dose of radiation is higher

Normal congruence angle (Merchant view) = 8.2°
Normal intercondylar groove angle (Merchant view) = 139° ± 6.3°
Lateral patellar subluxation more likely when the intercondylar angle approaches 150° or more

same criticism can be levelled against single views of patellar position within the femoral condylar notch, although much has been made of the congruency and tilting of the patella within this track (Figure 3.5). Recent studies with computerized tomography (CT) scanning now confirm that the radiographic appearance of the patella is inaccurately demonstrated by means of the skyline view, although this radiographic projection is useful in cases where an osteochondral fracture is suspected. One view of the patellofemoral joint may not in itself be sufficient and skyline views with the knee in varying degrees of flexion are essential.

Tunnel view

The intercondylar or 'tunnel' view of the knee shows whether a radio-opaque loose body is present in that region of the joint, and may give further information about the size and position of an osteochondritis dissecans involving the femoral condyle. The inferior pole of the patella may sometimes be shown clearly on the intercondylar view, as may an osteochondral fracture.

Oblique views of the knee are useful in revealing less obvious fractures, and anteroposterior and lateral 'stress' radiographs, preferably obtained when the patient is anaesthetized, are of value in recording ligament laxity or rupture. The use of an image intensifier and a video recorder will afford a dynamic assessment of the ligament injury which can then be stored.

Tomography

Tomograms of the knee can help to define lesions within the depth of the femoral condyles or proximal tibia, and lessen the artefacts caused by the superimposition of structures seen in the normal radiograph. Figure 9.16

(a,b) indicates the value of tomography in the case of a young man who presented with a painful knee. Routine investigations, including conventional radiography and arthroscopy, were normal. However, a tomogram revealed the pathological lesion, in this example a chondroblastoma.

Xeroradiography

Xeroradiography converts radiographic images to a blue-white detail based upon the photoconductor selenium, and gives a high-definition image of any soft-tissue changes in lesions such as neoplasm and infection. Soft-tissue shadows may be shown by abnormal swellings on the radiograph, and are best identified by comparison with the opposite knee. The uses of this technique are limited, however.

ARTHROGRAPHY

Arthrograms are produced by injecting a positive-contrast medium into the joint, Conray 280 giving good definition. Repeated tangential views of the medial and lateral menisci may reveal irregularities and tears within their structure (Figures 3.6 and 3.7), and the cruciate ligaments, articular surfaces of the knee and the size of any popliteal cyst can be defined (Stoker, 1980). Sometimes, synovial folds are demonstrated and one of them, the ligamentum mucosum, should be differentiated from the anterior cruciate ligament. Absence or rupture of the cruciate ligament is occasionally demonstrable.

Tears of the meniscus allow the contrast medium into the abnormal space, and if double-contrast is used there may be a filling defect. Vertical, longitudinal tears are readily seen, particularly if there is separation of the meniscal segments, but a transverse tear may be missed owing to the projection of the X-ray beam. Nevertheless arthrography affords a diagnostic rate of over 80% with such tears (Nicholas *et al.*, 1970; Ireland *et al.*, 1980).

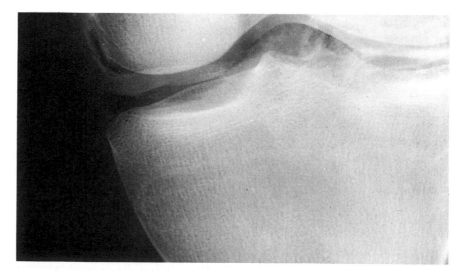

Figure 3.6 Arthrogram of a discoid lateral meniscus

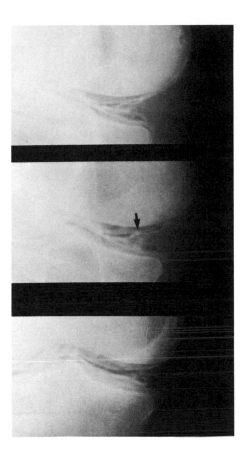

Figure 3.7 Arthrogram of a medial meniscal tear

Horizontal cleavage lesions of the meniscus usually show up clearly and are only difficult to interpret where there is a superimposition of other structures, such as in the posterolateral aspect of the knee where the popliteus tendon causes an artefact. The presence of degenerative changes throughout the knee may also make interpretation difficult, as may the combination of both vertical and horizontal tears within the meniscus. Lastly, a discoid meniscus, which is quite commonly the site of a tear, can be diagnosed by its bulk and rectangular outline.

Osteochondritis dissecans, with a separating fragment, and other irregularities of the articular cartilage, can be visualized by arthrography. However, the accuracy of diagnosis in cases of chondromalacia and early arthritis is less than 70%. In addition, abnormal structures within the knee, such as meniscal remnants, synovial tumours and loose bodies, can be identified, whereas they are often invisible on the standard radiograph as they are radiolucent. However, artefacts make the detection of synovial swellings and loose bodies difficult.

ARTHROSCOPY

Arthroscopic surgery of the knee is an integral part of orthopaedic practice (Tables 3.3–3.5), although it did not become established as a useful

Table 3.3 Use of arthroscopy

Meniscectomy	Anterior cruciate reconstruction	Arthrolysis
Meniscal repair	Lateral patellar release	Synovectomy
Removal of loose body	Resection of plica	Lavage/drainage
Articular cartilage excision/abrasion	Synovial biopsy	Tibial fracture reduction
Osteochondritis drilling/fixation	Excision of synovial lesion	Removal of implant

Table 3.4 Adjunctive use of diagnostic arthroscopy

Traumatic haemarthrosis	Osteochondritis
Patellar dislocation	Osteonecrosis
Chronic anterolateral laxity	Congenital limb anomalies
Arthritic knee prior to osteotomy	Skeletal dysplasia
Baker's cyst	

diagnostic aid until the early 1960s. Whereas clinical diagnosis of soft-tissue lesions in the knee offers an accuracy rate of approximately 65%, arthroscopy improves this figure to 80% or 90% and has the following advantages:

- More precise assessment of all three compartments of the knee
- Reduced morbidity from meniscal and patellofemoral surgery
- Facility for monitoring conditions affecting the knee

A patient admitted with a locked knee should be assessed by means of the arthroscope since a meniscal tear accounts for locking in less than half of the cases encountered (Gillquist *et al.*, 1977). For instance, a block to extension may be produced by ruptures of the anterior cruciate ligament or an anterior synovitis of the knee. In a proportion of cases no obvious abnormality is seen. Arthroscopic examination is particularly important in children where the clinical diagnosis is often erroneous.

The arthroscope affords a clear portrayal of the following conditions (McGinty and Matza, 1978; Dandy, 1981):

- Meniscal lesions, particularly vertical tears with displacement
- Anterior cruciate ligament rupture
- Synovial lesions (synovitis, synovial shelf impingement and synovial adhesions) (Patel, 1978)
- Articular cartilage wear and osteochondral fractures
- Loose bodies
- Fat-pad lesions and miscellaneous conditions such as haemangiomata

Certain loose bodies are hard to identify as they may be hidden in the recesses of the knee posteromedially, posterolaterally near the popliteus tendon, and in the periphery of the synovial cavity. Table 3.6 lists the sites in the knee where a good view may be difficult to obtain. These regions require the use of 30° and 70° telescopes and an alteration in technique before a diagnostic view can be obtained. Tears of the posterior cruciate ligament

Table 3.5 Complications of arthroscopy*

Complication	Percent
Haemarthrosis, haematoma	60.1
Infection	12.1
Thromboembolism	6.9
Anaesthetic problems	6.4
Instrument breakage	2.9
Reflex sympathetic dystrophy	2.3
Ligament tear	1.2
Fracture	0.6
Nerve injury	0.6
Other	6.9
	100.0

* Other complications include synovial fistula, compartment syndrome, portal wound tenderness and introduced drape fibres or talc (see Plate 37); articular scuffing occurs regularly but is hard to quantify.
From Small (1988), by permission.

Table 3.6 Potential arthroscopic 'blind spots'

Posterior recess including the posterior cruciate ligament
Posterior capsule
Posteromedial corner between the medial collateral ligament and the posterior horn of the medial meniscus
Beneath both menisci
Popliteus recess
Periphery of the patella and parts of the suprapatellar pouch

are difficult to identify, even with the 70° arthroscope, and partial tears of the anterior cruciate ligament may be missed if the synovial covering of the ligament appears intact. Probing or pulling on these structures with a blunt hook is of value in this context. Horizontal cleavage and peripheral tears of the menisci are not readily seen and the numerous causes of patellar pain are rarely apparent, partly because many of them are extra-articular and also because the mechanics of the patellofemoral joint cannot readily be assessed in the totally relaxed, anaesthetized patient. While the arthroscope usually gives a convincing picture of abnormalities which are obstructing knee movement, the diagnosis of chronic, painful conditions, unassociated with abnormal mechanical function, is difficult if not impossible.

The various portals of entry for the arthroscope are shown in Figure 3.8. Each surgeon will adopt procedures of his own choice and there are advantages to each approach. Certainly, no one site of insertion is superior and the surgeon should be prepared to utilize multiple views. The different types of arthroscopic telescopes are shown in Figure 3.9, together with some of the instruments which can be used.

A blunt hook is invaluable for probing structures under examination and allows undisplaced tears in the meniscus to be identified accurately,

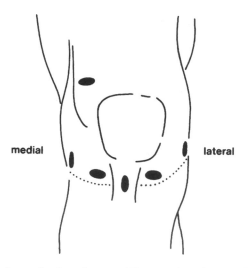

Figure 3.8 Portals of entry for the arthroscope. The anterolateral approach is generally preferred at the outset of the examination. Posterolateral and posteromedial portals are rarely required

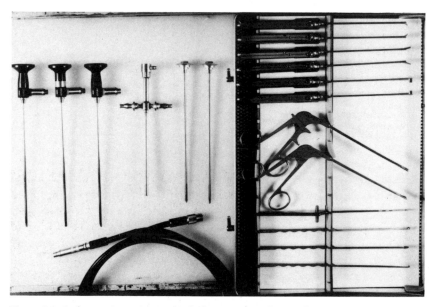

Figure 3.9 Arthroscopic equipment, including 0°,30° and 70° telescopes and fine instruments. Curved punch forceps and a sheathed blade are also of value

together with the stability of the meniscus. Cutting instruments are necessary if arthroscopic surgery is to be carried out and are combined with the use of grasping forceps with ratchet handles, rongeurs and biopsy forceps. Finally, the acquisition of a television monitor linked to a colour camera (see Plate 36) may assist in arthroscopic techniques and is a useful aid when instructing staff.

RADIOISOTOPE IMAGING

This technique is sensitive, but relatively non-specific (Table 3.7) (Lisbona and Rosenthal, 1977). It tends to overestimate the size of lesions in the region of the knee but does give dynamic information relating to the blood flow characteristics of a pathological process (Figure 3.10).

Table 3.7 Radioisotope imaging

Sensitivity	–	ability of a test to detect pathology
Specificity	–	ability of a test to detect normality
Accuracy	–	ability of a test to detect the true appearances

A variety of radioisotopes is concentrated in bone, and currently technetium 99m-labelled compounds (99mTc), such as methylene diphosphonate (MDP), are predominantly used for this purpose. After an intravenous injection, distribution of the isotope is identified on radiographic or polaroid film using a gamma camera to detect the radiation emitted. Bone can be scanned at various periods after injection of the isotope, a triple phase scan constituting: (1) images available after a half-minute, representing blood flow; (2) a blood pool phase, indicating vascularity; (3) a static phase obtained 2 hours after the bolus injection, defining the sequestration of the absorbed isotope.

A septic arthritis will produce increased uptake on both sides of a joint, whereas lesions within the bone will be concentrated on the affected side of the knee. Soft-tissue lesions tend to produce both increased flow and vascularity phases, with little bone absorption, whereas a synovitis increases isotope emission in all three phases.

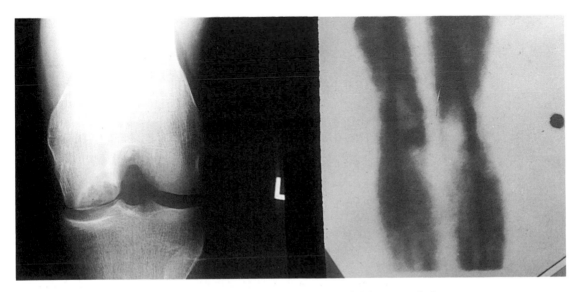

Figure 3.10 A radiographic lesion in the medial femoral condyle of the left knee (a) which is revealed as an area of increased uptake by radioisotope imaging (b)

When there is a chronic infection present, the triple phase scan may be negative if technetium is used, and in these instances a gallium 67-citrate (^{67}Ga) scan may be diagnostic. The gallium scan gives a more precise picture of local intraosseous involvement than technetium scintigraphy, but with the advent of CT and magnetic resonance (MR) imaging this technique is rarely used. Indium-labelled white cells may give a slightly more specific definition of an infective process than the triple phase technetium scan, but there is a minor increase in the dose of radiation. Bone tumours can be delineated by both the triple phase scan (Simon and Kirchner, 1980) and by monoclonal scans.

In conclusion, the following conditions cause increased uptake of radioisotope:

- Infection, including osteomyelitis
- Osteoarthritis where the features are detected earlier than with a radiograph
- Arthropathies, including rheumatoid arthritis and traumatic arthritis
- Tumours
- Fractures

Although bone scanning is sensitive to early pathological changes in bone it is a non-specific test and the diagnosis may still rest with the radiographic and histological features.

COMPUTERIZED TOMOGRAPHY

This sophisticated method, based upon X-rays, converts by computerization a succession of transverse radiographic sections of the knee to a three-dimensional view of the joint from 'within the tissues'. The technique is useful in assessing deeply-placed swellings, such as tumours, as there is little or no superimposition of other tissues upon the image under examination (Figure 3.11). A more accurate rendering of the patellofemoral joint can be obtained, and has shown how poorly the skyline radiographs define congruency of the patellofemoral joint and the various patellar shapes (Boven *et al.*, 1982).

Cruciate ligament tears can also be identified, and a combination of double-contrast arthrography with CT scanning adds greatly to the precision with which structures in the knee joint can be outlined. Soft-tissue, osseous and calcified masses can be seen, as may the three-dimensional patterns of fractures prior to decisions about internal fixation. CT scanning shows mineralization well, so that it offers superior images than MR in the detection of fracture, cortical destruction, intraosseous spread and soft-tissue calcification or ossification. The punctate calcification in chondromatous tumours and the reactive bone shell around an aneurysmal cyst are particularly clearly identified. CT scanning does not differentiate reliably between benign and malignant soft-tissue tumours, but their size and location can be defined and a lipoma (homogeneous fat density) can be distinguished from liposarcoma (heterogeneous fat density).

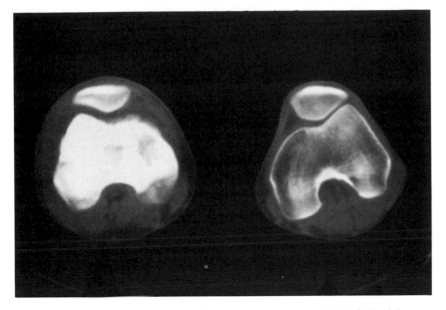

Figure 3.11 A computerized tomogram showing an osteosarcoma of the left distal femur

VENOGRAPHY AND ARTERIOGRAPHY

The injection of radioisotope contrast materials into the veins and arteries of the leg is diagnostic in a number of conditions. Deep venous thrombosis can be reviewed accurately, and can be differentiated from a ruptured popliteal cyst, both conditions producing calf pain and swelling.

Arteriography is an essential investigation in the severely injured limb with compromised vascularity. The site of arterial injury, whether a laceration, thrombosis or embolism, can be identified with precision and appropriate surgical treatment instituted. This facility is also valuable in the treatment of certain tumours with extensive arteriolar and capillary networks. Thus the arteriogram will outline the size and spread of the neoplastic mass, allowing appropriate surgery to be planned. If a tumour such as an aneurysmal bone cyst or haemangioma merits embolization, arteriography will define the feeder vessels and the pattern of venous drainage, and the characteristics of arteriovenous malformations, aneurysms and fistulae can be defined.

MAGNETIC RESONANCE IMAGING

Magnetic and electromagnetic fields interact with tissues according to their different densities, producing measurable signals (Table 3.8 and Figures 3.12–3.20). MR imaging does not define cortical changes as readily as CT scanning and oedema produces an abnormal signal which may be confusing. But axial, coronal and sagittal displays are highly accurate and help to detect intraosseous and extraosseous pathology (Berquist, 1989).

Table 3.8 High-intensity signal

Grade I	Central and globular
Grade II	Primarily linear, not extending to surface
Grade III	Linear and extending to surface

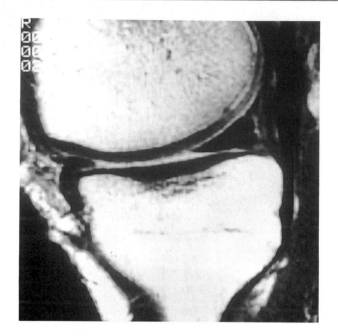

Figure 3.12 A normal meniscal outline

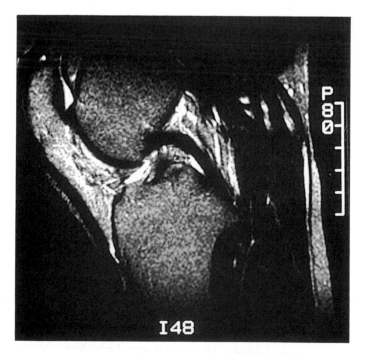

Figure 3.13 An intact posterior cruciate ligament

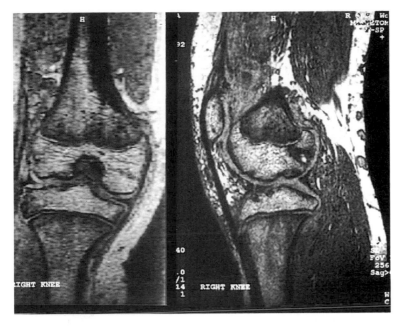

Figure 3.14 Repeated bleeds into the knee from an arteriovenous malformation have produced irregularity of the articular cartilage and the formation of bone cysts

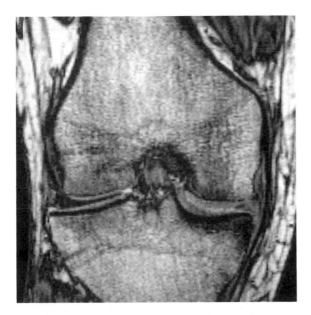

Figure 3.15 A discoid lateral meniscus

The anatomical relationships of soft-tissue masses and the delineation of vascular structures are so good that angiography is little indicated. Lipogenic tumours produce higher intensity signals than muscle on T_1- and T_2-weighted images, whereas other tumours have low signals on T_1-weighted images and high signals on T_2-weighted images. Malignancy

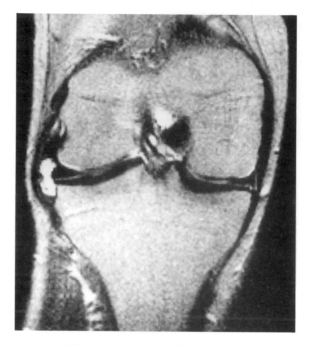

Figure 3.16 A peripheral meniscal cyst

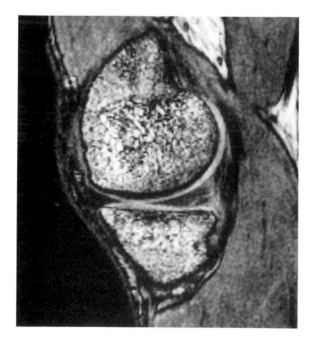

Figure 3.17 A meniscal tear

produces a more heterogeneous mass and may be surrounded by the high signal of oedema on the T_2-weighted scan. MR imaging is superior to CT scanning in the evaluation of most soft-tissue tumours and lesions about the knee.

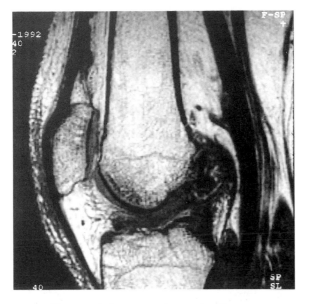

Figure 3.18 A torn anterior cruciate ligament

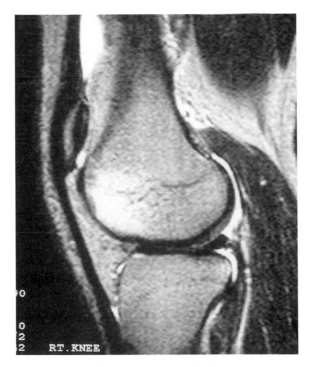

Figure 3.19 A bone bruise

Meniscal tears and cruciate ruptures are detected with an accuracy of between 75% and 95%t (Fischer *et al.*, 1991), although a negative MR scan does not rule out intra-articular (Raunest *et al.*, 1991) or peri-articular pathology. Arthroscopy may miss grade II (incomplete) tears (Table 3.8),

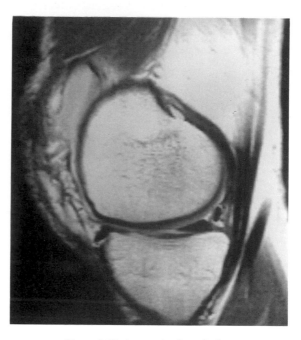

Figure 3.20 A posterior loose body

although many of these may heal. Quinn and Brown (1991) considered that the error rate between the two investigations also reflected the experience of the surgeon and the difficulties inherent in visualizing the posterior horn of the menisci. Inner third tears are often minor and asymptomatic so that the surgeon may discount them as significant. It should also be appreciated that grades I and II lesions may not progress appreciably with time (Dillon *et al.*, 1991) and that stable lesions are common and consistent with satisfactory knee function. More alarmingly, progression in the signal intensity is seen as a result of a season playing American football (Reinig and McDevitt *et al.*, 1991) although some lesions may subsquently heal.

Previous meniscectomy, meniscal repair and degenerative change affect the MR scan, making its clinical relevance less obvious. It may well be that bone marrow and articular cartilage lesions inevitably develop in conjunction with anterior cruciate disruption or other injuries (Speer *et al.*, 1991). Changes are also detectable in chondromalacia patellae (Hodler and Resnick, 1992), although Spiers *et al.* (1993) considered that the MR scan afforded a low sensitivity of only 18% for articular cartilage lesions.

The cruciate ligaments are structures of low signal intensity although the anterior, in contrast to the posterior, is not invariably seen on sagittal scans. A torn anterior cruciate ligament presents with an undulating or irregular anterior margin, high signal intensity within its substance on T_2-weighted images, or a gap. Oedematous intercondylar soft tissue is seen with acute tears (Vahey *et al.*, 1991) and the knee laxity may cause anterior bowing of the posterior cruciate ligament. Chronic tears show up with disruption of the contour, atrophy or absence, although scar tissue may bridge across or the anterior cruciate remnant may adhere to the posterior cruciate ligament.

After reconstruction increased signals (T_1- and T_2-weighted) may still be consistent with an intact neoligament, although gross focal changes and a wavy outline suggest laxity or rupture. Impingement produces a high-intensity signal in the distal one-third of the graft.

It may well be that scanning does pick up continuing pathology within the substance of a sutured meniscus and Negendank *et al.* (1990) showed the presence of meniscal degeneration in the asymptomatic, contralateral knee of patients with meniscal symptoms.

RADIONUCLIDE SCINTIGRAPHY

Single photon emission computerized tomography (SPECT) is a useful means of ruling out lesions in the knee which might give rise to anterior knee pain (Murray *et al.*, 1990). Arthroscopic intervention becomes unnecessary and sympathetic blockage may be considered in those with increased uptake on the scan, despite a lack of the features normally associated with reflex sympathetic osteodystrophy (Butler-Manuel *et al.*, 1992). True chondromalacia patellae can be detected accurately by combining T_1-weighted (proton-density) images with T_2-weighted images (McCauley *et al.*, 1992).

THERMOGRAPHY

Thermographic assessment of the anterior knee pain syndromes provides colourful but non-specific appearances (see Plate 47). The investigation is helpful in monitoring the response of an arthropathic knee to medical or surgical treatment. During the early, vasodilatory phase of reflex sympathetic dystrophy (see page 197), temperature changes of 2°C or more are recorded and may help in the earlier diagnosis and management of this troublesome condition. However, the investigation is principally recording from surface blood vessels and its role in knee conditions is therefore somewhat limited and rarely improves upon careful clinical examination.

ULTRASOUND

Although ultrasound is diagnostically useful in outlining structures within the abdomen and pelvis, and the unstable hip joint in the neonate, its use in the knee is limited. Soft-tissue tumours and effusions or cysts can be detected, and the investigation is both cheap and non-invasive.

CYBEX DYNAMOMETRY

Muscle power in the hamstrings and quadriceps can be measured by means of the Cybex dynamometer or KinCom apparatus. The effort produced by the patient is calculated in terms of work output and thus the recovery from injury and the power in various muscle groups can be monitored regularly (see Chapter 10).

EXERCISE TESTS

Simple walking tests are of value in assessing basic gait patterns and loss of walking speed. Measurements of stride length and cadence can be obtained easily, and the patient may be filmed during walking. More sophisticated gait analysis laboratories will define the characteristics of each walking pattern, and these results can be combined with the use of force-plate studies of the weightbearing foot, thus giving a more dynamic but at times very complex picture of the mechanics of walking or running.

References

Berquist, T.H. (1989) Magnetic resonance imaging of musculoskeletal neoplasms. *Clin. Orthop.*, **244**, 101–118

Boven, F., Bellamans, M.A., Geurts, J. *et al.* (1982) The value of computed tomography scanning in chondromalacia patellae. *Skeletal Radiol.*, **8**, 183–185

Butler-Manuel, P.A., Justins, D. and Healtey, F.W. (1992) Sympathetically mediated anterior knee pain: scintigraphy and anaesthetic blockade in 19 patients. *Acta Orthop. Scand.*, **63**, 90–93

Dandy, D.J. (1981) *Arthroscopic Surgery of the Knee*, Churchill Livingstone, Edinburgh

Dillon, E.H., Pope, C.F., Joki, P. *et al.* (1991) Follow-up of Grade II meniscal abnormalities in the stable knee. *Radiology*, **181**, 849–852

Fischer, S.P., Fox, J.M., Del Pizzo, W. *et al.* (1991) Accuracy of diagnosis from magnetic resonance imaging of the knee. A multi-center analysis of one thousand and fourteen patients. *J. Bone Joint Surg.*, **73A**, 2–10

Gillquist, J., Hagber, G. and Oretorp, N. (1977) Arthroscopy in acute injuries of the knee joint. *Acta Orthop. Scand.*, **48**, 190–196

Hodler, J. and Resnick, D. (1992) Chondromalacia patellae : commentary. *Am. J. Roentgenol.*, **158**, 106–107

Hughston, J.C. (1968) Subluxation of the patella. *J. Bone Joint Surg.*, **50A**, 1003–1026

Ireland, J., Trickey, E.L. and Stoker, D.J. (1980) Arthroscopy and arthrography of the knee. A critical review. *J. Bone Joint Surg.*, **62B**, 3–6

Laurin, C.A., Dussault, R. and Levesque, H.P. (1979) The tangential investigation of the patellofemoral joint. *Clin. Orthop. Rel. Res.*, **144**, 16–26

Lisbona, R. and Rosenthal, L. (1977) Observations on the sequential use of ^{99m}Tc-phosphate complex and ^{67}Ga imaging in osteomyelitis, cellulitis and septic arthritis. *Radiology.*, **123**, 123–129

McCauley, T.R., Kier, R., Lynch, K.J. *et al.* (1992) Chondromalacia patellae : diagnosis with MR imaging. *Am. J. Roetngenol.*, **158**, 101–105

McGinty, J.B. and Matza, R.A. (1978) Arthroscopy of the knee. Evaluation of an out-patient procedure under local anaesthetic. *J. Bone Joint Surg.*, **60A**, 787–789

Merchant, A.C., Mercer, R.L., Jacobsen, R.H. and Cool, C.R. (1974) Roentgenographic analysis of patellofemoral congruence. *J. Bone Joint Surg.*, **56A**, 1391–1396

Murray, I.P.C., Dixon, J. and Kohan, L. (1990) SPECT for acute knee pain. *Clin. Nucl. Med.*, **15**, 828–840

Negendank, W.G., Fernandez, F.R., Heilbrun, L.K. and Tietge, R.A. (1990) Magnetic resonance imaging of meniscal degeneration in asymptomatic knees. *J. Orthop. Res.*, **8**, 311–320

Nicholas, J.A., Freiberger, R.H. and Killeran, P.J. (1970) Double-contrast arthrography of the knee. Its value in the management of two hundred and twenty-five knee derangements. *J. Bone Joint Surg.*, **52A**, 203–220

Patel, D. (1978) Arthroscopy of the plica – synovial folds and their significance. *Am. J. Sports Med.* **6**, 217–225

Quinn, S.F. and Brown, T.F. (1991) Meniscal tears diagnosed with MR imaging versus arthroscopy : how reliable a standard is arthroscopy. *Radiology*, **818**, 843–847

Raunest, J., Oberle, K., Leonhert, J. *et al.* (1991) The clinical value of magnetic resonance image in the evaluation of meniscal disorders. *J. Bone Joint Surg.*, **73A**, 11–16

Reinig, J.W., McDevitt, E.R. and Ove, P.N. (1991) Progression of meniscal degenerative changes in college football players : evaluation with MR imaging. *Radiology*, **181**, 255–257

Simon, M.A. and Kirchner, P.T. (1980) Scintigraphic evaluation of primary bone tumours. Comparison of technetium-99m phosphonate and gallium citrate imaging. *J. Bone Joint Surg.*, **62A**, 758–764

Small, N.C. (1988) Complications in arthroscopic surgery performed by experienced arthroscopists. *Arthroscopy*, **4**, 215–221

Smillie, I.S. (1980) *Diseases of the Knee Joint*, 4th edn, Churchill Livingstone, Edinburgh

Speer, K.P., Spritzer, C.E., Goldner, J.L. and Garrett, W.E. Jr. (1991) Magnetic resonance imaging of traumatic knee articular cartilage injuries. *Am. J. Sports Med.*, **19**, 396–402

Spiers, A.S.C., Meagher, T., Ostlere, M. *et al.* (1993) Can MRI of the knee affect arthroscopic practice? *J. Bone Joint Surg.*, **75B**, 49–52

Stoker, D.J. (1980) *Knee Arthrography*, Chapman and Hall, London

Vahey, T.N., Broome, D.R., Kayes, K.J. *et al.* (1991) Acute and chronic tears of the anterior cruciate ligament : differential features at MR imaging. *Radiology*, **181**, 251–253

4
Paediatric injuries

CHARACTERISTICS – AETIOLOGY – PATELLAR INSTABILITY –
ACUTE HAEMARTHROSIS – LIGAMENT INJURIES – MENISCAL
TEARS – OSTEOCHONDRAL LESIONS – MISCELLANEOUS
CONDITIONS

Trauma produces the same types of injury in the child as in the adult (Backx *et al.*, 1989) but the patterns are age-related. The 5-year-old is more likely to suffer from the exacerbation of malalignment (Figure 4.1; see also Plates 26 and 27) or torsional abnormalities, affecting the patellofemoral mechanism and the growth plate, whereas the 15-year-old is prone to ligament tears and avulsions. Overuse syndromes and 'growing pains' more typically affect the older child.

Joint laxity is associated with a number of inherited conditions (Table 4.1) and may result in symptoms without an obvious precipitating injury. Similarly, familial hypermobility and persistent femoral anteversion adversely affect patellar tracking, yet it is often this very group of children who are adept athletically and thus promote patellar instability. Ligament sprains and osteochondral lesions occur with greater stress and will recur if muscle tone is not restored. During maturation the problems associated with malalignment and laxity may lessen, although a proportion of patients continue to suffer from the patella or the tibial collateral ligament.

The last important characteristic is the fact that the symptomatic knee acts as a conduit for lumbar spine and particularly hip pathology in the growing child, and may also be the target organ in a child with emotional problems, including the individual who finds that the pressures of a competitive sport have become too great. Mild spastic hemiplegia, spinal cord lesions, limb length discrepancy and hip disorders such as transient synovitis, Perthes' disease, development dysplasia and slipped upper

Table 4.1 Conditions associated with ligament laxity

Down's syndrome	Achondroplasia
Ehlers–Danlos syndrome	Nail-patella syndrome
Marfan's syndrome	Ellis–van Creveld syndrome
Turner's syndrome	Osteogenesis imperfecta

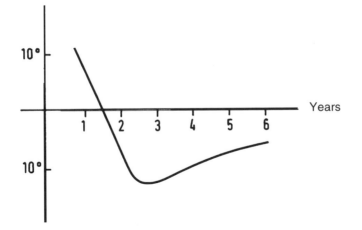

Figure 4.1 *The mean tibiofemoral angle changes from varus to valgus during early childhood*

femoral epiphysis must be excluded by careful clinical examination, radiographic review and imaging, as appropriate.

Table 4.2 shows the symptoms which presented in 1000 consecutive cases referred with knee complaints to a clinic in Edinburgh during 1983–89 (Macnicol, 1994). In a proportion with patellar pain and those with non-specific synovitis the term 'irritable knee' is appropriate, provided that referred pain has been ruled out and the joint feels warm and intermittent swelling is reported. The onset of symptoms could be attributed to sports in 60% (Table 4.3).

Arthroscopic intervention is required in a relatively small proportion, and is rarely indicated for the anterior knee pain and patellar instability groups. However, since MR imaging may be poorly tolerated, and chronic synovitis and anxiety may retard progress with physiotherapy, arthroscopic review is recommended in some children with patellar pain and apparent

Table 4.2 Knee disorders in 1000 consecutive cases

Patellar pain	61%
Osgood–Schlatter's disease	17%
Patellar dislocation	11%
Synovitis	4%
Meniscal lesion	2%
Other	5%

Table 4.3 Sports producing knee symptoms, in decreasing order of frequency

Soccer *	Skiing *
Rugby *	Swimming
Athletics	(Highland) dancing
Gymnastics *	Other (mountain biking, etc.)

* More likely to cause avulsion injuries.

Table 4.4 Knee disorders encountered in 100 consecutive arthroscopies

Meniscal lesions	27
Osteochondritis dissecans	26
Synovitis	20
Normal	18
Cruciate pathology	5
Chondromalacia patella	4

restriction of the passive range of movement (Table 4.4; see also Plate 25). As in the adult, the procedure reduces the synovitis and the aching pain, the child and parents are reassured that no major pathology is present and in every case the symptoms have relented after vigorous physiotherapy has been reinstituted, often as an inpatient for the first few days postoperatively. Only in the smaller child is the use of small-diameter arthroscopes or needlescopes necessary (Plate 37) and distension of the knee is usually perfectly adequate to allow safe use of the adult arthroscope and sheath.

PATELLAR INSTABILITY

Although the patellofemoral mechanism is the major site of problems in childhood, most of the symptoms do not develop as a result of sports alone. The exceptions to this rule are those children where repetitive exercises induce overuse syndromes : gymnastics, swimming and athletics are most likely to produce problems. The extensor mechanism is vulnerable along its full length and avulsion injuries are relatively common, including Sinding–Larsen–Johansson syndrome, avulsion marginal fractures and tibial apophyseal fractures (Figure 4.2). Most of these injuries settle with rest from the sport, coupled with physiotherapy and supportive strapping. Splintage with casts should be avoided, even in painful and recurrent Osgood–Schlatter's condition. In approximately one-third of children, the sport will no longer be pursued, and only a further third will return to the same level of competitive activity.

Patellar instability is often associated with a relatively short quadriceps mechanism, and the degree to which this is present may be classified in terms of diminishing severity from congenital dislocation (see Figure 2.2), to habitual dislocation and finally to the recurrent or intermittent dislocation and subluxation which affect the adolescent (Macnicol and Turner, 1994). Associated skeletal abnormalities are shown in Figure 7.1, but as these usually cannot be altered, at least during a particular stage in childhood, therapy consists of stretching the quadriceps and improving inner range (vastus medialis) power. If quadriceps elongation is not achieved, relative patella alta persists (Micheli *et al.*, 1986) and may be worsened by lateral release (Hughston and Deese, 1988). Hence realignment must only be considered after a careful assessment of the mechanics of the paediatric patellofemoral mechanism (Goa *et al.*, 1990).

In the athletic child lateral patellar release is all that has been necessary when physiotherapy fails (Dandy and Griffiths, 1989). More extensive procedures are rarely indicated and should be avoided when there is gross

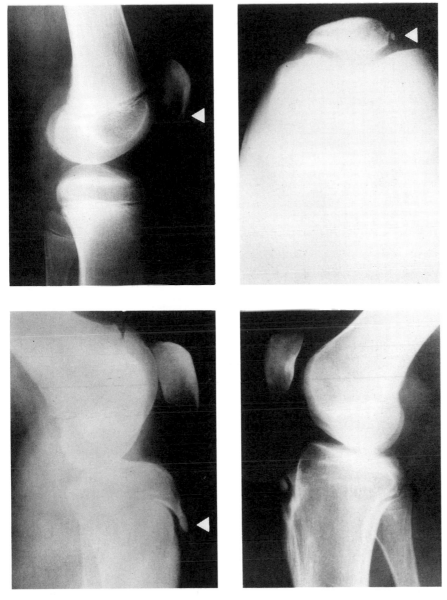

Figure 4.2 *Different sites of stress can be detected radiographically*

ligament laxity and when the patella dislocates in a sinusoidal manner, both in extension and flexion (see Figure 7.8). Pain at rest is another relative contraindication to patellar realignment which must always be preceded by a diagnostic arthroscopy.

ACUTE HAEMARTHROSIS

Sudden swelling of the traumatized knee is relatively rare in children playing sports, and usually indicates the formation of a haemarthrosis secondary to patellar dislocation (with or without osteochondral fracture),

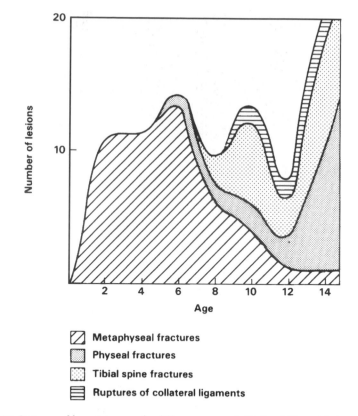

Metaphyseal fractures
Physeal fractures
Tibial spine fractures
Ruptures of collateral ligaments

Figure 4.3 Patterns of knee injury at the different stages of childhood (From Skak et al., 1987)

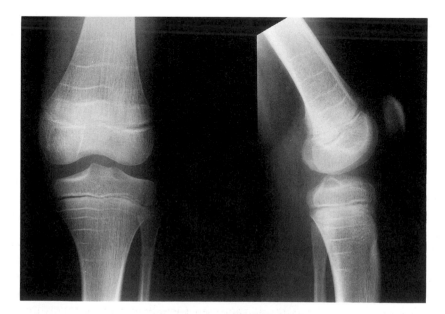

Figure 4.4 Growth arrest (Harris) lines produced by the stress of skiing every winter

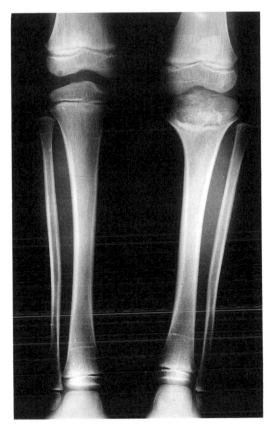

Figure 4.5 Proximal tibial growth arrest produced by an injury when mountain biking

ligament avulsions and tears, and other rare pathologies (Plates 45 and 46). Injuries to the cruciate and medial ligaments were also found to account for half the cases of haemarthrosis by Eiskjaer *et al.* (1988). Arthroscopy reveals that haemorrhage occurs from the synovial invaginations and peripheral folds as well as from the cruciate ligament stump or from osteochondral fractures. Young children are not immune to significant ligament ruptures. Waldrop and Broussard (1984) reported a mophead (isolated) anterior cruciate ligament tear in a child of 3 years, and Joseph and Pogrund (1978) encountered a medial collateral ligament tear in a 4-year-old child (after a road traffic accident).

Severe ligament disruption is more likely in later childhood and adolescence, the younger child suffering metaphysial fractures, ligament avulsions and growth plate disturbance (Figure 4.3). However, occult ligament injury probably occurs in all cases of avulsion injury, and growth plate disturbance may produce subtle signs radiographically (Figure 4.4), rather than overt physeal arrest (Figure 4.5). The haemarthrosis may promote a persisting synovitis or a mild form of reflex sympathetic dystrophy, both of which will prolong morbidity. Direct synovial injury from a blow over the anteromedial aspect of the knee during games occasionally produces a subsequent medial shelf syndrome, or patellar tendonitis.

LIGAMENT INJURIES

Medial collateral ligament

Medial collateral ligament sprains and tears are managed conservatively, as described by Indelicato (1983) in the adult. It is wise to carry out an arthroscopy or MR scan in order to rule out concomitant injury, looking particularly for anterior cruciate ligament rupture, meniscal lesions or osteochondral fractures. Splintage is best avoided, but if examination under anaesthesia reveals significant medial gapping and an appreciable suction sign, a moulded backshell or a hinged brace may be appropriate, together with protected weightbearing for approximately 4 weeks. Commercially available canvas backshells are best avoided as they are poorly tolerated by the child and often ill-fitting.

Anterior cruciate ligament

Avulsion of the tibial eminence by the anterior cruciate ligament has attracted much attention recently after Meyers and McKeever (1970) reported a series of 47 cases. Their grades I and II injuries (Figure 4.6) did well with conservative treatment in 80%. They recommended open reduction for the type III, fully avulsed fragment which is often irreducible. This was recognized by Zaricznyj (1977) who graded the type III injury as follows: (a) complete fragment pull off but no rotation; (b) complete displacement with rotation. A type IV avulsion was also described, consisting of a larger, comminuted fracture extending into the medial and lateral tibial plateaux.

Accurate reduction involves the replacement of one or other wing of the fragment below the anterior meniscal horns and the intermeniscal ligament, and it is suggested that internal fixation may then be unnecessary. But the risk of leaving the fragment proud, and the anterior cruciate ligament unnecessarily lax, is a real one.

If splintage is felt to be appropriate the knee should not be extended fully as this may lift the fragment upwards by tautening the ligament. Equally, there is the view that extension (but not hyperextension) will allow the femoral condyle to push the tibial fragment into place (Robinson and Driscoll, 1981). Splintage for 8 weeks is sufficient to ensure union of the

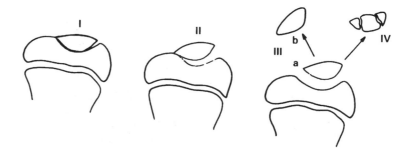

Figure 4.6 *The grading of intercondylar eminence avulsion fractures*

fragment if it has been anatomically replaced. Rehabilitation is slow, with restriction of full extension and flexion for up to a year. Residual laxity is often apparent later, and Grove *et al.* (1983) considered the results of non-operative treatment to be unsatisfactory.

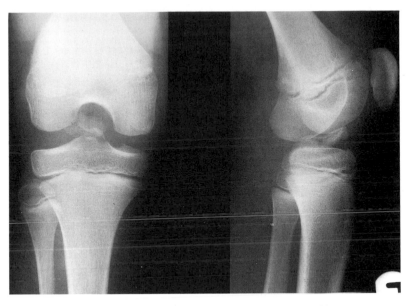

Figure 4.7 A type IIIB fracture which was irreducible

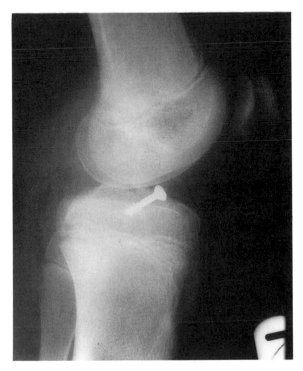

Figure 4.8 Reduction and fixation of the fragment with an intra-epiphysial screw

Open reduction and fixation, often possible by an arthroscopically assisted technique, should ensure the best outcome. Insertion of an intra-epiphysial screw is usually safe if it is inserted obliquely (Figures 4.7 and 4.8), and this alignment is usually necessary if the knee is being held in only partial flexion in order to relax the anterior cruciate ligament injury. Operative treatment is also advisable if collateral ligament tears and meniscal detachment are suspected (Lisser and Weiner, 1991). Mid-substance tears are probably underdiagnosed, and it is likely that some ligament disruption coexists with avulsion fractures, whether tibial or femoral.

Ligament reconstruction is occasionally indicated, for it is now realized that conservative treatment or acute repair is as fruitless as it is in the adult. However, early diagnosis of anterior cruciate ligament rupture should allow a substantial portion of the natural ligament to be incorporated in any reconstruction. The damaged ligament is sutured alongside a semitendinosus autogenous graft. This is left attached distally and is only placed in a bone tunnel through the proximal tibial growth plate if the patient is within two years of maturity. In the relatively rare case involving a younger child, reinforcement of the natural ligament is possible by routing the graft over the upper surface of the epiphysis, tunnelling proximal to the physis (Henning, 1992). Femoral attachment at the isometric point is achieved by screw or staple fixation, avoiding a full bone tunnel. The 'over the top' route is preferred by some surgeons, and avoids concern about distal femoral growth plate damage.

Graft protection is ensured for a minimum of 3 months, with limited weightbearing and supervised movement of the knee, allowing virtually full extension from the outset but controlling the power applied through the quadriceps group. There is a natural tendency towards a 'quadriceps avoidance gait' so that bracing is of limited value. Proprioception and confidence are built up progressively and full sporting activity is usually allowed at the anniversary of the operation. The results of treatment for tibial eminence avulsion are often disappointing. Smith (1984) found that half the patients in his series suffered from pain or instability on average 7 years later and Gronqvist *et al.* (1984) considered that late instability was proportional to the age of the child when injured. The results of anterior cruciate ligament reconstruction have not been reported after a sufficiently long-term review (McCarroll *et al.*, 1988) but it is hoped that the depressing natural history of anterior cruciate deficiency will be altered favourably.

Posterior cruciate ligament

This injury is rare (Mayer and Micheli, 1979) at approximately 10% of the frequency of anterior cruciate ligament rupture. It is important to recognize the significance of posterior cruciate ligament rupture, for the long-term disability is persistent and virtually impossible to overcome later. The mechanism is usually a blow over the upper shin when playing football or impacts from mountain biking or skiing. If bone has been avulsed (Figures 4.9 and 4.10), reattachment of the anchor point is achieved with an intra-epiphysial screw and rehabilitation is reasonably rapid, provided that there has been no delay in treatment. Associated knee injuries are rare, although the posterolateral structures may be damaged.

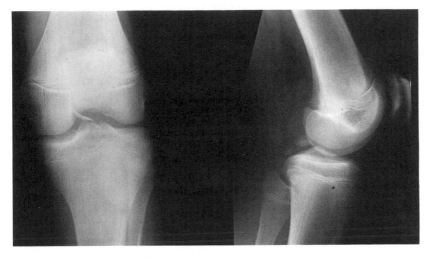

Figure 4.9 Avulsion of the femoral attachment of the posterior cruciate ligament

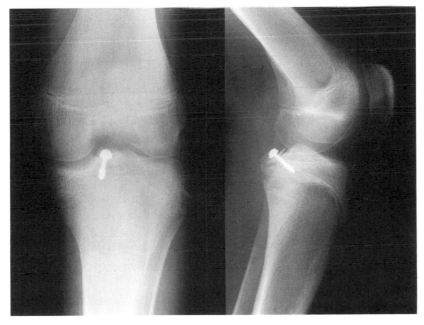

Figure 4.10 Internal fixation of the fragment with a lag screw and washer

Lateral complex avulsion

Avulsion of the biceps and popliteus tendons results from major varus stress (Figure 4.11). The iliotibial tract is usually spared, but repair is always advised when there is significant gapping and a suction sign over the posterolateral joint line, since the tendons quickly retract and become irreparable. Peroneal nerve traction lesions may coexist in the adult but are unusual in the child.

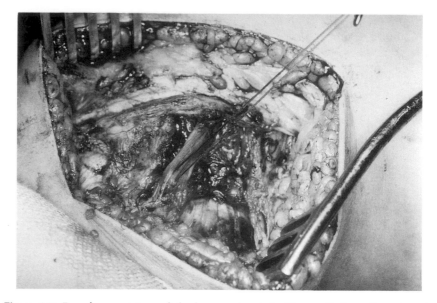

Figure 4.11 *Forced varus injury of the knee produced significant soft-tissue disruption; the avulsed biceps tendon (attached to a stay suture) will retract if left unrepaired*

After surgery the knee is protected in slight flexion using a cast in the younger child or a brace in the adolescent. Residual laxity is common but may lessen if the child has several years of skeletal growth ahead.

MENISCAL TEARS

The discoid anomaly is relatively common in the younger child, causing one form of the snapping knee. However, it is uncommon to find it as an acute meniscal problem, tears developing slowly over a period of months. The classical, and reasonably normal discoid meniscus, covering much of the lateral tibial condyle, develops a tear in its medial edge. Partial excision of the damaged segment is achieved arthroscopically or through a mini-arthrotomy, allowing the rim to function relatively normally. However, it should be remembered that the dynamic attachments of the discoid meniscus are also abnormal so that mild symptoms are likely to persist.

If the Wrisberg form of anomaly is encountered (see Plate 44), complete excision may be necessary, although this decision should be deferred for as long as possible. Preservation of meniscal tissue remains the goal, particularly in the growing child. Meniscal repair is appropriate for displacing 'bucket handle' tears and peripheral splits, although healing of menisci undoubtedly occurs as a natural process without surgical intervention if a peripheral separation or longitudinal split is stable and the knee is protected. Radial tears are rare in childhood, although they may affect the lateral meniscus in the adolescent. The lesion should be saucerized in an attempt to prevent the tear from spreading peripherally, and if a peripheral cyst develops this can be decompressed through the line of cleavage of the tear.

Minor lesions of the meniscus are produced by impingement or subluxation. This is a product of meniscal mobility and the lax mesentery of the meniscotibial ligament is akin to the recognized problem of patellar hypermobility. A blush of inflammatory tissue similar to early pannus is seen overlying the anterior meniscal horn (see Plate 38) and there is a concurrent articular cartilage lesion. These meniscal impingements are seen in sports demanding repetitive stresses, such as gymnastics or dancing, and may be associated with articular cartilage debris from overuse.

Meniscectomy in childhood is known to produce significant later problems in a high proportion of cases (Zaman and Leonard, 1981; Menzione *et al.*, 1983; Abdon *et al.*, 1990). Partial meniscectomy and successful meniscal repair should improve the prognosis, although there are no long-term reports of the outcome after these procedures as yet. An analysis of the literature dealing with the effects of discoid meniscal partial excision also confirms that there are no grounds for complacency (Ikeuchi, 1982; Hayashi *et al.*, 1988; Vandermeer and Cunningham, 1989; Aichroth *et al.*, 1991).

OSTEOCHONDRAL LESIONS

The exact cause of osteochondritis dissecans is debatable, and trauma may be no more than a promoting factor. In the pre-teenage child the appearance of the lesion may be developmental, either vascular or secondary to an aberration of ossification. The symptoms of pain, clicking or locking and sometimes swelling generally occur with sport, yet in only half of the cases can a true sporting injury be implicated.

If the lesion is confined to the classical site (see Figure 9.13) it is more likely to heal. Arthroscopic review or MR scanning is indicated, as it is important to confirm that the articular cartilage remains intact over the lesion. The majority of children can safely be followed up with restriction of sport advised until symptoms have disappeared and there is radiographic evidence of healing. At arthroscopy, synovial adhesions may be found attached to the lesion and these are best released, with a postoperative emphasis upon regaining movement since the extremes of flexion and extension are regularly lost.

When the fragment is shown to be separating, and this is more common in adolescence, when the lesion is more extensive, or at an unusual site, then fixation by the Herbert screw, two retrograde K wires or a small fragment, counter sunk AO screw is advised. Fibrin glue is too weak to secure the lesion and polyglycolic acid pegs may cause a chronic inflammatory reaction. The base of the lesion should be freshened so that the inserted fragment does not stand proud, and if the condylar bed appears to be avascular it is more appropriate to excise the fragment unless it is very large. If the lesion fails to unite after fixation, the fragment should be removed before adaptive changes occur over the tibial surface in contact. Even the loss of large osteochondritic fragments may be consistent with satisfactory function since the defect fills slowly with fibrocartilage. Long-term reviews suggest that arthritic changes are advanced by 10 years, but there is no convincing evidence that replacement of the fragment significantly alters the natural history.

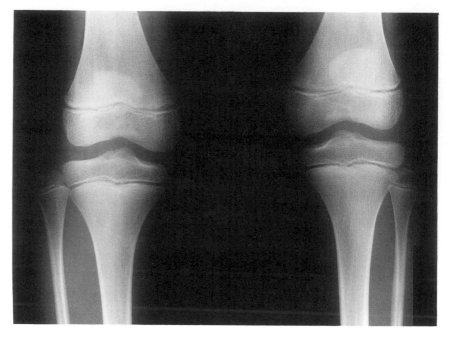

Figure 4.12 *Anterolateral subluxation of the right proximal tibiofibular joint with overgrowth of the fibula*

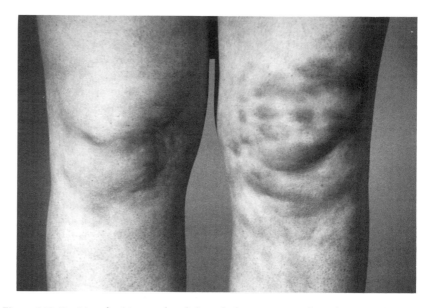

Figure 4.13 *Factitious bruising produced through the anterior window of a canvas knee splint*

True osteochondral fractures occur in association with patellar dislocation; these are differentiated by their bleeding base and acute onset. Cartilaginous flaps and small separated fragments do not usually merit replacement, but osteochondral fragments over 1 cm in diameter should be fixed in place and usually unite.

MISCELLANEOUS CONDITIONS

When assessing the child with a symptomatic knee following injury, generalized and local pathology should always be considered, in addition to the typical injuries described. Developmental conditions, bleeding disorders, atopy (asthma, hay fever and eczema) and synovial lesions must all be considered. Injuries to the growth plate may be subtle or overt, and in some cases the symptoms coincide with a sporting injury but are primarily acquired from a different disease process (see Figure 9.5). Therefore it is vital to take a full history and examine the child completely, even after the most obvious sporting injury. Proximal tibiofibular subluxation (Figure 4.12 and Plate 31) and referred pain from the hip are two conditions where errors are regularly made.

The child under psychological pressure from the parents, the coach or the sport, may suffer emotionally. In these instances the knee may become the target organ of complaint (Figure 4.13) and minor malfunctions may be much exaggerated. Counselling or cessation of the sport may be the only means of resolving the conflict. Remember also that every active child is 'sporting' in the sense that regular and repetitive exercise occurs with play. When the demands of growth combine with an active lifestyle and the pressures of organized sport, the knee is frequently the site of first complaint.

References

Abdon, P., Turner, M.S., Pettersson, H. *et al.* (1990) A long-term follow-up study of total meniscectomy in children. *Clin. Orthop.*, **257**, 166–170

Aichroth, P.M., Patel, D.V. and Marx, C.L. (1991) Congenital discoid lateral meniscus in children; a follow-up study and evolution of management. *J. Bone Joint Surg.*, **73B**, 932–936

Backx, F.J.G., Erich, W.B.M., Kemper, A.B.A. and Verbeek, A.L.M. (1989) Sports injuries in school-aged children : an epidemiologic study. *Am. J. Sports Med.*, **17**, 239–240

Dandy, D.J. and Griffiths, D. (1989) Lateral release for recurrent dislocation of the patella. *J. Bone Joint Surg.*, **71**, 121–125

Eiskjaer, S., Larsen, S.T. and Schmidt, M.B. (1988) The significance of hemarthrosis of the knee in children. *Arch. Orthop. Trauma Surg.*, **107**, 96–98

Goa, G.-X., Lee, E.H. and Bose, K. (1990) Surgical management of congenital and habitual dislocation of the patellae. *J. Pediatr. Orthop.*, **10**, 255–260

Gronqvist, H., Hirsch, G. and Johansson, L. (1984) Fractures of the anterior tibial spine in children. *J. Pediatr. Orthop.*, **4**, 465–467

Grove, T.P., Miller, S.J. III, Kent, B.E. *et al.* (1983) Non-operative treatment of the torn anterior cruciate ligament. *J. Bone Joint Surg.*, **65A**, 184–188

Hayashi, L.K., Yamaga, H., Ida, K. *et al.* (1988) Arthroscopic meniscectomy for discoid lateral meniscus in children. *J. Bone Joint Surg.*, **70A**, 1495–1500

Henning, C.E. (1992) Anterior cruciate ligament reconstruction with open epiphyses. In: *Knee Surgery Current Practice* (eds Aichroth, P.M. and Cannon, W.D.), Martin Dunitz, London, pp. 181–185

Hughston, J.C. and Deese, M. (1988) Medial subluxation of the patellae as a complication of lateral retinacular release. *Am. J. Sports Med.*, **16**, 383–388

Ikeuchi, H. (1982) Arthroscopic treatment of discoid lateral meniscus : technique and long-term results. *Clin. Orthop.*, **167**, 19–28

Indelicato, P.A. (1983) Non-operative treatment of complete tears of the medial collaeral ligament of the knee. *J. Bone Joint Surg.*, **65A**, 323–329

Joseph, K. and Pogrund, H. (1978) Traumatic rupture of the medial ligament of the knee in a four year old child : case report and review of the literature. *J. Bone Joint Surg*, **60A**, 402–403

Lisser, S. and Weiner, L.S. (1991) Ligament injuries in children. In: *Ligament and Extensor Mechanism Injuries of the Knee; Diagnosis and Treatment* (ed. Scott, W.N.) Mosby, St Louis

McCarroll, J.R., Retting, A.C. and Shelbourne, D.K. (1988) Anterior cruciate ligament injuries in the young athlete with open physes. *Am. J. Sports Med.*, **16**, 44–49

Macnicol, M.F. (1995) Sports injuries of the knee in children. *Int. Orthopaedics*, **3**, 27–36

Macnicol, M.F. and Turner, M.S. (1994) *The Knee*. In: *Children's Orthopaedics and Fractures* (eds Benson, M.K.D., Fixsen, J.A. and Macnicol, M.F.), Churchill Livingstone, Edinburgh, pp. 484–485

Mayer, P.J. and Micheli, L.J. (1979) Avulsion of the femoral attachment of the posterior cruciate ligament in an 11-year-old boy : case report and review of the literature. *J. Bone Joint Surg.*, **61A**, 431–432

Menzione, M., Pizzutillo, P.D., Peoples, A.B. *et al.* (1983) Meniscectomy in children: a long-term follow-up study. *Am. J. Sports Med.*, **11**, 111–115

Meyers, M.H. and McKeever, F.M. (1970) Fracture of the intercondylar eminence of the tibia. *J. Bone Joint Surg.*, **41A**, 209–222

Micheli, L.J., Slater, J.A., Woods, E. *et al.* (1986) Patella alta and the adolescent growth spurt. *Clin. Orthop.*, **213**, 159–162

Robinson, S.C. and Driscoll, S.E. (1981) Simultaneous osteochondral avulsion of the femoral and tibial insertions of the anterior cruciate ligament. *J. Bone Joint Surg.*, **63A**, 1342–1343

Skak, S.V., Jensen, T.T., Poulsen, T.D. *et al.* (1987) Epidemiology of knee injuries in children. *Acta Orthop. Scand.*, **58**, 78–81

Smith, J.B. (1984) Knee instability after fractures of the intercondylar eminence of the tibia. *J. Pediatr. Orthop.*, **4**, 462–466

Vandermeer, R.D. and Cunningham, F.K. (1989) Arthroscopic treatment of the discoid lateral meniscus : results of long-term follow-up. *Arthroscopy*, **5**, 101–109

Waldrop, J.I. and Broussard, T.S. (1984) Disruption of the anterior cruciate ligament in a three-year-old child. *J. Bone Joint Surg.*, **66A**, 1113–1114

Zaman, M. and Leonard, M.A. (1981) Meniscectomy in children : results in 59 knees. *Injury*, **12**, 425–428

Zaricznyj, B. (1977) Avulsion fracture of the tibial eminence : treatment by open reduction and pinning. *J. Bone Joint Surg.*, **59A**, 1111–1114

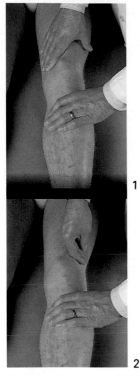

1

2

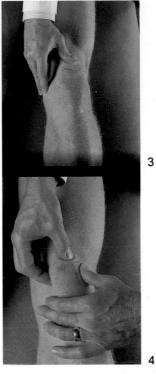

3

4

5(a)

5(b)

Plate 1 Synovial fluid is swept up into the suprapatellar pouch by the flat of the right hand; the return of fluid into the medial patellar hollow will be seen in a moderate effusion, if the patient is not obese

Plate 2 When the effusion is minor, the lateral gutter and patellar pouch must be emptied by using the back of the right hand, again sweeping upwards

Plate 3 The patellar restraint test produces forcible compression of the patella against the femoral sulcus when the quadriceps contracts

Plate 4 The retropatellar surface and synovial margin can be palpated if the knee is relaxed and extended

Plate 5 Tapping the femoral condyle with the middle finger elicits local tenderness in osteochondritis dissecans, infection and other skeletal lesions

Plate 7 The fibular head should be palpated for tenderness or swelling, and to detect proximal tibiofibular subluxation (comparing one side to the other)

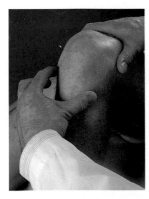

Plate 6 Joint line tenderness suggests meniscal pathology and should be elicited precisely, using the index finger with the knee flexed to a right angle

6

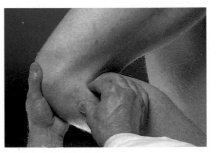

7

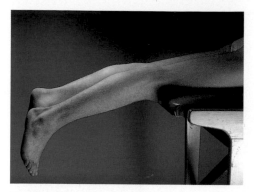

Plate 8 The prone-lying test on a firm surface identifies minor restrictions of extension (as in the locked knee) and hyperextension (after ligament rupture)

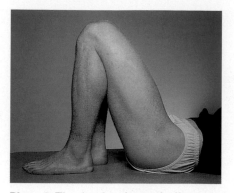

Plate 9 The heel-to-buttock distance is the best measure of minor losses of knee flexion, commonly seen in posterior compartment pathology

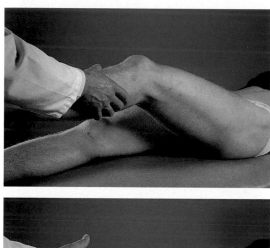

a

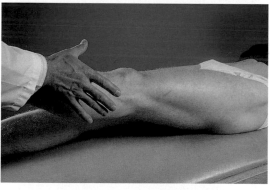

b

Plate 10 The bounce test assesses whether the knee extends fully by means of its 'screw home' action. Anterior meniscal tears, loose bodies and chondral lesions impede the sense of the knee dropping out straight as the right hand releases its support (a & b).

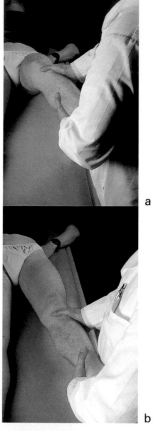

a

b

Plate 11 The medial collateral structures are assessed by applying a valgus force with the knee 20° flexed (a) and then extended (b). If the joint opens medially in extension the injury is significant, probably involving the anterior cruciate ligament and/or the posterior capsule

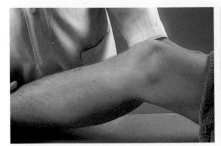
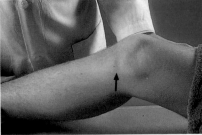

Plate 12 A medial joint line suction sign indicates a grade II tear with a definite firm end point

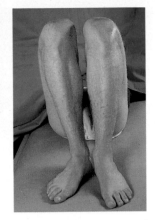

Plate 14 If the thigh is supported under the examiner's knee, anteroposterior and collateral laxity can be assessed accurately as the patient relaxes

Plate 13 Increased external rotation of the tibial secondary to post-traumatic laxity of the right knee (if the knee is locked, rotation is reduced)

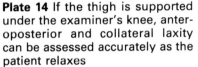

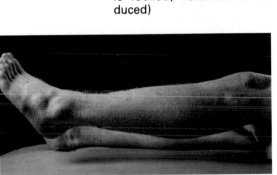

Plate 15 With a plinth or the examiner's forearm to support the thigh, dynamic measurement of anterolateral laxity is often possible during active knee extension

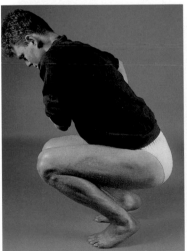
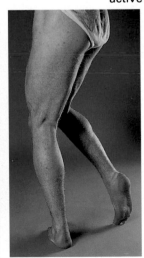

Plate 16 Squatting and 'duck-waddling' prove impossible in the presence of a displacing meniscal tear

Plate 17 Internal and external rotation on the weightbearing leg elicits discomfort at the site of a meniscal lesion and apprehension if rotatory laxity is present

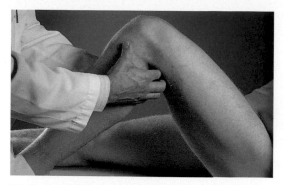

Plate 18 The anterior drawer test fixes the foot and assesses the knee in 90° of flexion after checking that the hamstrings are relaxed

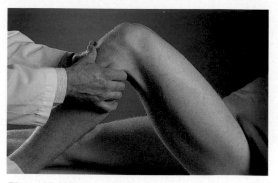

Plate 19 When anterior laxity is present the hamstrings will involuntarily contract

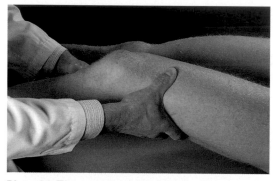

Plate 20 The standard Ritchey–Lachman test (see p 27)

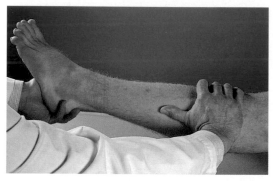

Plate 21 Anterolateral subluxation can be produced with axial pressure from the left hand and the right hand exerting a valgus and anterior force against the fibula

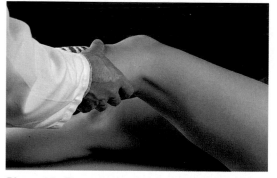

Plate 22 The pivot shift may be demonstrated from the flexed position to extension

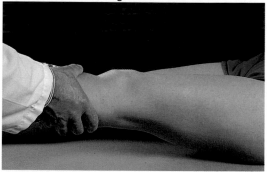

Plate 23 With the knee in extension, the subluxed lateral tibial condyle will be reduced by a return to the flexed position (see also Figures 2.11–2.13)

5

Ligamentous injuries

MEDIAL LIGAMENT TEARS – ANTERIOR CRUCIATE
LIGAMENT TEARS – POSTERIOR CRUCIATE LIGAMENT
TEARS – LATERAL LIGAMENT COMPLEX INJURIES

Over the last decade no topic in orthopaedic management has evoked greater interest than knee ligament tears. The knee is vulnerable to soft-tissue injury because it is an unconstrained hinge placed at a site where collisions and twisting stresses are readily sustained at sport and during everyday activity.

The integrity of the normal knee is maintained by the two cruciate ligaments centrally and a succession of structures around the periphery of the joint. Medially, the two laminae of the tibial collateral ligament and the posteromedial capsular corner of the knee are reinforced by the pes anserinus group (sartorius, gracilis and semitendinosus) and the semimembranosus (see Figure 1.2). On the lateral side the fibular collateral ligament and arcuate ligament posteriorly are augmented by the tendons of popliteus and biceps femoris. Further forward the anterolateral femorotibial ligament and iliotibial band (see Figure 1.3) reinforce the capsule.

Anteriorly the quadriceps mechanism is a vital, dynamic stabilizer while the sturdy posterior capsule, including its oblique popliteal ligament, is augmented by the semimembranosus, popliteus and gastrocnemius tendons (see Figure 1.8). The joint surfaces and menisci impart little stability to the joint which is therefore highly dependent upon the passive and dynamic supports described.

In the child, avulsion of the skeletal attachment of the ligament is more likely until the age when the growth plate is fusing. Low-velocity trauma in the adult usually results in a mid-substance rupture, but it is also clear that the ligament avulsion produced by greater force inevitably causes a varying degree of soft-tissue disruption. Noyes et al. (1974) assessed the pathological changes in stressed ligaments during experiments in primates and found that ligament failure often preceded tibial eminence avulsion by the anterior cruciate ligament, with a 57% incidence at a slow loading rate and a 28% incidence at a faster loading rate. Tearing of the ligament is usually more substantial when assessed throughout its length microscopically, involving the neural network as well as collagen fibres, elastin and

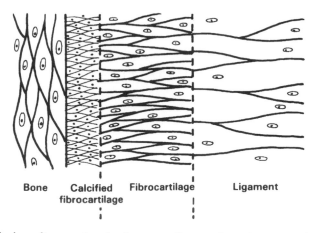

Figure 5.1 *The bone–ligament junction forms a resilient gradient of progressively more elastic tissue from bone (left) to calcified fibrocartilage, unmineralized fibrocartilage and then ligament (right)*

capillaries. An intact synovial sheath may disguise the extent to which the ligament is ruptured.

The bone–ligament junction is an important structure, allowing a controlled gradient between hard and soft tissue. Bone, with a matrix of principally chondroitin sulphate, blends with a layer of calcified fibrocartilage (detectable histologically as a basophilic blue line of mineralization) and then a wider zone of fibrocartilage (Panni *et al.*, 1993). The type I collagen fibrils of 25–300 mm diameter are anchored in this resilient zone of fibrocartilage which acts as a 'stretching brake' (Figure 5.1). The bone–ligament junction is 3–4 times as strong as the central part of the ligament, and in the normal situation it is unlikely to yield. However, fibrous tissue replaces the fibrocartilage layer when artificial ligament replacements are used. This envelope, similar to the fibrous tissue layer around the cement mantle of an arthroplasty, has relatively poor tensile properties so that the attachment of Dacron directly to bone is physiologically unsatisfactory. Panni *et al.* (1993) showed that the Kennedy ligament augmentation device (LAD), wrapped in tendinous connective tissue, produced less fibrous tissue than an uncovered artificial ligament, although the layer was always thicker than that seen with the bone–patellar tendon–bone autograft bedded into bone tunnels.

Ligament injuries are arbitrarily divided into three grades:

- First-degree sprain in which there may be micro-tears within the structure of the ligament, but the strength of the ligament is clinically unimpaired
- Second-degree sprain in which there is a partial tear of the fibres composing the ligament, such that some lengthening and subsequent laxity is evident (5–10 mm more than the opposite side)
- Third-degree sprain in which the ligament is torn across completely and offers no stability to the knee (more than 10 mm of excess laxity, and with no feeling of an 'end point')

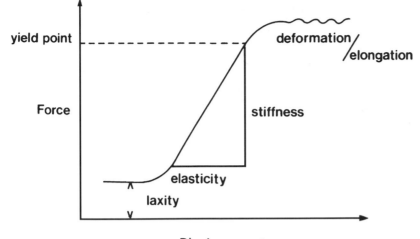

Figure 5.2 *If a force (newtons) is progressively applied to a ligament, as shown on the ordinate, the slack is first taken up before the ligament stretches under load in a way that is dictated by its modulus of elasticity. As long as the yield point is not exceeded, the ligament will return to its prestressed state. When deformation (irreversible elongation) occurs, by definition the ligament is beginning to tear. The extent of this plastic change is proportional to the load (strain) applied. The mean maximum failure load (yield point) is approximately 1500 N for the anterior cruciate ligament, double this for the posterior cruciate ligament and never more than half this for autogenous grafts*

Avulsion injuries occur between bone and the zone of calcified fibrocartilage. This junction is more vulnerable in the child and adolescent, and is somewhat akin to the growth plate.

Although a great deal has been written about the passive, restraining action of the ligaments (Figure 5.2), this is only one part of their function. It is clear that all ligaments are supplied with sensory nerve endings, and

Table 5.1 Proprioception is provided by a variety of intra-articular sensors

Type	Location	Function
Golgi tendon organ (fusiform corpuscle)	Ligaments, meniscal horns	Dynamic mechanoreceptor (high threshold)
Ruffini (globular corpuscle)	Ligaments, menisci, capsule, fat-pad	Static and dynamic mechanoreceptor
Pacinian (conical corpuscle)	Ligaments, menisci, capsule, fat-pad	Dynamic mechanoreceptor (low threshold)
Free nerve endings: thinly myelinated unmyelinated*	All articular tissues except cartilage	Nociceptors or non-nociceptive mechanoreceptors

* Neuropeptide release causes inflammation (and later osteoarthritis) by stimulating the proliferation of synoviocytes.

Table 5.2 Classification of articular receptors

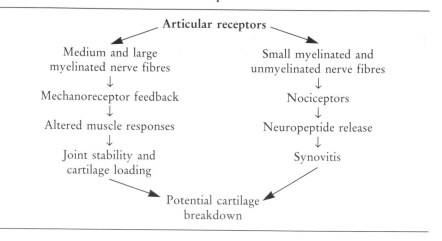

these mechanoreceptors can be identified on the surfaces of the ligament (Tables 5.1 and 5.2). Thus, the ligaments provide a very important sensory function role, feeding afferent impulses to the central nervous system and thereby setting up reflexes which inhibit potentially injurious movements of the knee (see Figure 1.1).

MEDIAL LIGAMENT TEARS

The medial ligament not only prevents valgus deviation of the tibia below the femur, but also prevents the tibia from rotating externally under the femoral condyles. A knowledge of this second function is important, as the tests used to assess the medial ligament and associated supporting structures are devised to show any pathological forward and outward movement of the medial tibial condyle. There will therefore not only be an increased tilting of the knee, but also a rotation which is termed anteromedial laxity if in excess of that found in the other knee.

It has already been mentioned that the knee should be assessed in extension and in a little over 10° of flexion, the latter affording a more precise assessment of the medial structures alone, whereas the former tests the integrity also of the posterior capsule and the cruciate ligaments. A further assessment is carried out with the knee in 90° of flexion. Not only should an abnormal degree of external tibial rotation be noted when performing the anterior drawer test, but also an increase in forward glide of the medial plateau of the tibia will occur if the foot is externally rotated after an initial assessment with the tibia and foot in the neutral position (see Chapter 2).

Pathology

The site of the medial ligament tear can often be identified by palpation and there may be associated bruising after 12 or 24 hours. Significant disruption of the medial collateral ligament will result in tearing of not only the more superficial tibial collateral portion, but also the deep and capsular component (Figure 5.3). This will allow a suction sign to develop, whereby the increased tilting of the tibia on the femur draws in the soft tissues as the joint opens up abnormally on the medial side (see Plates 45 and 46). The leaking of blood from the disrupted capsule will be manifest by loss of the normal haemarthrosis after such injuries. Instead, there will be a boggy ecchymosis over the medial side of the knee and valgus stress will cause the medial side to hinge open if the patient is anaesthetized (Figure 5.4).

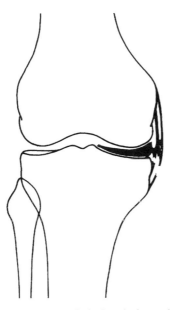

Figure 5.3 *The medial ligaments are closely linked with the medial meniscus*

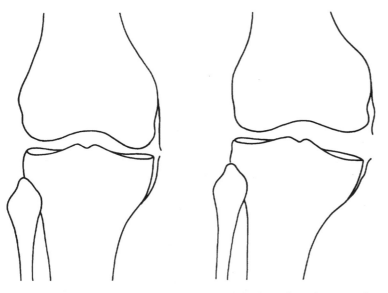

Figure 5.4 *Valgus stress will open up the medial side of the knee, dependent upon the extent of the soft-tissue injury and the degree of protective muscle spasm*

Treatment

First-degree sprains are treated by the local application of ice, compression and occasionally strapping. Early movement is encouraged by physiotherapy, although pain will prevent a normal range of movement or full weightbearing initially. Associated tears of the medial meniscus or anterior cruciate ligament are unlikely, yet it is occasionally necessary to investigate the knee further by means of MR scanning and possibly arthroscopy if an obstructive lesion appears to be present. Meniscal tears, chondral flaps and osteoarthritis may impede recovery, and intermittent symptoms may persist for over a year.

Second-degree tears are treated in similar fashion, although there is a greater incidence of associated injury. Investigation includes the standard biplanar radiographs, and an examination under anaesthesia including arthroscopy is often advised in order to assess the pathological valgus laxity and concurrent injuries more accurately. Strapping and protected weightbearing may be helpful for up to 6 weeks, and quadriceps and hamstring drill should be supervised for several months. With time the abnormal laxity should reduce as interstitial healing proceeds; however, a mild degree of residual laxity is common and splintage of the knee in flexion is sometimes advisable during the first 2–4 weeks.

Complete or third-degree tears can be managed conservatively since surgical intervention does not appear to hasten recovery (Indelicato, 1983). This applies particularly to tears above the joint line, unless avulsion of the adductor tubercle is present, when reattachment is a relatively simple procedure. In the acute phase, pain limits activity and a 2–4-week period of backshell splintage and protected weightbearing is necessary.

Mid-portion tears of the ligament are more disruptive since the meniscotibial ligament is involved. Arthroscopy will allow an assessment of the meniscal rim and posteromedial capsule. If the meniscus is stable there is no advantage from surgical repair, but if the meniscus is dislocated a peripheral repair should be attempted (see Chapter 6). Direct suture of the middle or lower thirds of the tibial collateral ligament is ineffectual, although reefing and augmentation with the pes anserinus or a medial strip of patellar tendon has been advocated when associated tears of the anterior cruciate ligament merit intervention. In general, medial collateral injury is now managed conservatively unless specific features make surgery advisable. In particular, combined anterior cruciate ligament (ACL) and medial ligament tears provide a relative indication to repair or reconstruct both structures, particularly when valgus laxity in extension persists after ACL reconstruction. However, in women or less athletic individuals there is an increased risk of postoperative stiffness so that medial ligament repair should not be considered (Shelbourne and Basle, 1988).

ANTERIOR CRUCIATE LIGAMENT TEARS

These tears present acutely or chronically, and in the acute lesion the other knee ligaments may be clinically normal. Amis and Scammell (1993) have found that anterior displacement of the tibia sufficient to disrupt the ACL will leave the collateral ligaments unstretched, although the posteromedial and posterolateral structures will be stretched. Non-contact deceleration and sudden, inward twisting of the knee may also cause 'isolated' ACL rupture, the patient experiencing a popping sensation in approximately half the cases. Hyperflexion with the tibia internally rotated may rupture either or both cruciates, and forced hyperextension will cause varying severities of ACL tear. Combined injuries occur from impact over the side of the knee; the medial collateral structures are torn, followed by the ACL which angulates against the lateral femoral condyle. There may be associated meniscal injuries, patellar subluxation and osteochondral fractures.

Early examination will reveal anterolateral laxity but later swelling and spasm will obscure this. The Lachman test (see Chapter 2) identifies this laxity more readily than the 90° drawer test since the restraining effect of the posterior meniscal horns is reduced and the collateral structures are relatively lax. In time, the secondary restraints slacken under the increased load, although the knee may compensate so that disabling instability and a positive pivot shift are not invariable. The patient will adapt by using a 'quadriceps-avoidance' gait (Berchuck *et al.*, 1990), reducing the magnitude of flexion and extension. Kinematic studies show these changes during walking or jogging, but activities employing greater flexion of the knee, such as climbing or descending stairs, are not appreciably affected. Even after surgical reconstruction this altered pattern may persist, similar to the altered gait adopted after pes anserinus transfer (Perry *et al.*, 1980).

Undoubtedly the most disabling symptom experienced by the individual convalescing after ACL rupture is the sense of giving way or buckling, induced unexpectedly when the weightbearing knee is rotated. Concordance between this symptom of instability and a positive pivot shift test is high, although the test may be pronounced negative by the inexperienced examiner and is often difficult to elicit in the conscious patient who actively guards against the subluxation.

The long-term prognosis after ACL rupture is difficult to predict, partly because each patient represents a different combination of aspirations, secondary laxity and morphological features such as leg alignment, lateral tibial contour and muscle tone (Macnicol, 1989), and partly because the orthopaedic literature on the subject is conflicting. Most studies are retrospective, including different patient groups and varying patterns of associated injury. Furthermore, there is still a lack of uniform preoperative and postoperative grading.

Overall, one-third of patients appear to compensate sufficiently to return to sport, often to quite a high level of competition, and it is difficult to predict the outcome at the time of the acute injury . Hughston's comment should be kept in mind: 'I see many more disabled knees resulting from anterior cruciate repair, augmentation and reconstruction than I see with absence of the anterior cruciate ligament' (Hughston and Barrett, 1983).

If the knee fails to compensate, chronic anterolateral laxity may initiate a remorseless train of events leading to meniscal tears, articular cartilage wear and progressive osteoarthritis (Figures 5.5 and 5.6). The radiographic changes include:

- Avulsion, prominence or spurring of the intercondylar spines
- Narrowing of the intercondylar notch

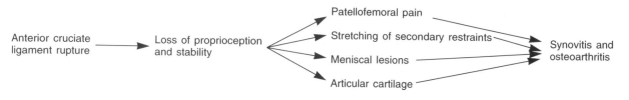

Figure 5.5 *Rupture of the anterior cruciate ligament may initiate a remorseless train of events leading to osteoarthritis*

- The Segond fracture (lateral capsular sign) (Figure 3.3b)
- Notching of the lateral femoral condyle posterior to Blumensaat's line (similar to the glenohumeral Hill–Sachs lesion)
- Arthritic change, initially in the lateral compartment

Although the osteoarthritis may stabilize the knee, lateral meniscal tears and chondral lesions generally conspire to produce symptoms. If pain persists at times other than when the knee suddenly subluxes, it may be inadvisable to consider surgical reconstruction of the ligament. Arthroscopic intervention should be limited to meniscal and articular cartilage tears. However, when pain and effusions are short-lived, occurring immediately after the episode of buckling, stabilization of the knee is important. Reconstruction has been shown to decrease the incidence of later meniscal tears from approximately 60% to 10% (Balkfors, 1982) and meniscal repair is more likely to succeed although it is still less effective than in the normal knee (Cannon and Vittori, 1992).

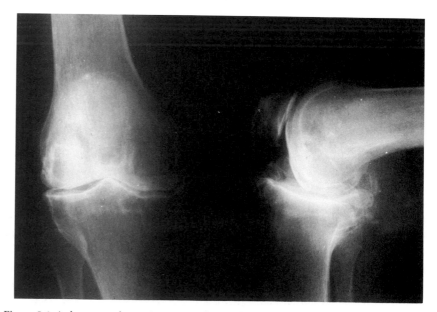

Figure 5.6 *A documented anterior cruciate ligament tear 20 years before produced these gross arthritic changes*

The evolution of ACL reconstruction

During the nineteenth century a number of surgeons recognized the features of ACL rupture and attempted to brace the knee. Bonnet of Lyons published a textbook in 1845 which described proximal ACL avulsion, haemarthrosis and tibial subluxation, and both he and Stark of Edinburgh (Stark, 1850) used hinged braces for the unstable knee. Georges Noulis, a Greek surgeon, published a description of the Lachman test in 1875 and Segond, a French surgeon, published in 1879 the pain, pop and swelling characteristic of ACL rupture, together with the fracture that bears his name (Pässler, 1993). Annandale (1885) was the first to record a successful meniscal repair, while Hey–Groves (1917) wrote extensively on the subject of cruciate ligament repair. Attempts with tendon substitutes, fascia lata, the meniscus and black silk were usually only partially satisfactory and the reconstructions tended to stretch with time.

Palmer (1938) and Smillie (1978) published seminal work on the soft-tissue injuries involving the knee and now knee reconstructive surgery is widely practised in Europe, North America and the Far East. A bewildering number of retrospective reports dealing with the proposed advantages of ACL repair and reconstruction are only gradually leading to any consensus about the management of this condition, and many of the recommendations remain controversial and poorly researched. However, some of the principal issues will be addressed:

- Is there a convincing reason to repair or reconstruct all acute injuries?
- What are the relative indications for chronic reconstruction?
- Is there any evidence to show which form of reconstruction is more likely to succeed?
- What happens to autografts in the long term, and will the knee continue to benefit from surgery after 10 years?
- Is there a place for artificial ligaments and allografts?
- Should extra-articular reinforcement be used to augment the intra-articular graft?
- Is there evidence to suggest that the intra-articular graft should be supported with a ligament augmentation device?

Acute intervention

In children, adolescents and athletes under the age of 30 years, reattachment of the ACL is appropriate, particularly those cases of intercondylar eminence avulsion where the fragment is irreducible (see Figure 4.7). If the growth plate is open, drill holes through the physis should be avoided unless the child is within a year or two of maturity.

If ligament tears are dealt with early, suturing may be sufficient. However, it is usually difficult to gain sufficient ligament length and therefore augmentation with tendon or patellar retinaculum is advisable (Jonsson *et al.*, 1990). Augmentation is essential for mid-substance, 'mop end' tears (Engebretsen *et al.*, 1990), but in both instances preservation of the remnants of the ACL is recommended unless the soft-tissue bulk in the intercondylar notch is excessive, producing impingement or friction. The semitendinosus graft is ideal for the reconstruction and can be used as a double loop.

Acute ACL reconstruction is also indicated in patients with an associated grade III collateral ligament rupture or with a repairable meniscal tear. Where osteochondral fracture or major, multidirectional laxity is encountered, early surgical intervention may be justifiable but an increased risk of stiffness from fibrosis has been reported (Sgaghone *et al.*, 1993) and there may be a case for waiting a few weeks until the acute haemarthrosis has resorbed (Shelbourne *et al.*, 1991). Partial ACL ruptures are generally more significantly torn than may appear on probing, but a conservative approach with surgical follow-up is appropriate in all but the top level athlete since the morbidity from surgery is appreciable (Sandberg *et al.*, 1987).

Indications for chronic reconstruction

A conservative approach is advised initially after arthroscopy or MR scanning has confirmed the presence of a chronic ACL deficiency. However, the therapeutic effect of exercise and of bracing is often short-lived (see Chapter 10) and the patient returns later, stating that the knee is still troublesome. Motivation and general fitness are important attributes if the reconstruction is to succeed, and the physiotherapist who has been treating the patient is an important ally in reaching the correct decision about surgical intervention.

There should be negligible arthritic change radiographically, although articular cartilage degeneration is almost inevitable in the athlete with chronic anterolateral laxity. Patients over the age of 40 years are rarely considered for operation, but in selected cases the results are gratifying. A severely decompensated knee, affected by regular buckling and hyperextension, cannot be ignored if conservative measures fail, and repeated effusion or the development of meniscal tears are indications for surgery. However, persistent pain is of concern as it may be worsened by cruciate ligament reconstruction.

Obviously each surgeon will develop his own threshold for intervention, but it is important to avoid being too readily persuaded by patients if clinical features suggest they are unsuitable, and a second opinion is worth while in borderline cases. Generally speaking, it is accepted that one-third of those who present will continue to manage conservatively, particularly if their sporting aspirations are curtailed, and a further third merit immediate reconstruction owing to the decompensation. The middle third may cope with encouragement but may require surgery at a later date. Measurement of the degree of anterolateral laxity using the KT-1000 arthrometer (see Figure 10.4) has been found to help with this decision (Daniel, 1990) and the outcome depends upon patient selection, surgical technique and the postoperative rehabilitation.

Method of reconstruction

In acute reconstruction a semitendinosus graft appears to give as much stability as the patellar tendon, despite its relative weakness (Figure 5.7). In chronic reconstruction the bone–patellar tendon–bone autograft has been looked upon as the gold standard, although its advantage over hamstring grafting is not clear cut (Marder *et al.*, 1991; Aglietti *et al.*, 1992), the results

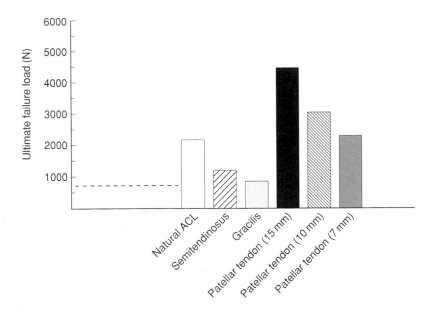

Figure 5.7 *The strength of ACL substitutes. The dotted line indicates the maximum strength of graft fixation initially*

at 2 years being similar apart from greater donor site morbidity with patellar tendon harvesting. Patellar symptoms complicate the use of the patellar graft more frequently than with semitendinosus (Sachs *et al.*, 1989), although the strength of fixation of the former may be greater. By 8 weeks in the goat model, failure of the graft shifts from its site of attachment to the midsubstance of the tissue (Holden *et al.*, 1988). Clancy *et al.* (1981) showed in Rhesus monkeys that the graft remained weak for at least a year, and recent clinical studies confirm that laxity usually persists to some degree.

Long-term benefits of reconstruction

Any improvement in knee stability must be set against the complications and failures of ligament reconstruction. In addition to graft rupture (partial or complete), loss of movement, effusions, wound infection and septic arthritis, patellar symptoms, tenderness at tunnel sites and over metal implants and muscle hernia are recorded problems. Reviews of the results of ACL reconstruction are rarely sufficiently extensive in time and detail (Johnson *et al.*, 1984) since remodelling of the graft is very slow. The inserted tissue is known to remain mechanically inferior for several years (Ballock *et al.*, 1989) and is dependent upon placement (Figure 5.8), physiological loading and adequate revascularization for its survival. Impingement between the graft and the femur in extension (Figure 5.9) (Howell and Taylor, 1993), loss of fixation and an inadequate return of proprioception imperil the graft throughout the first few years of function. Thereafter a low grade synovitis, particularly from breakdown products, may promote the very degenerative changes that the procedure is designed to prevent.

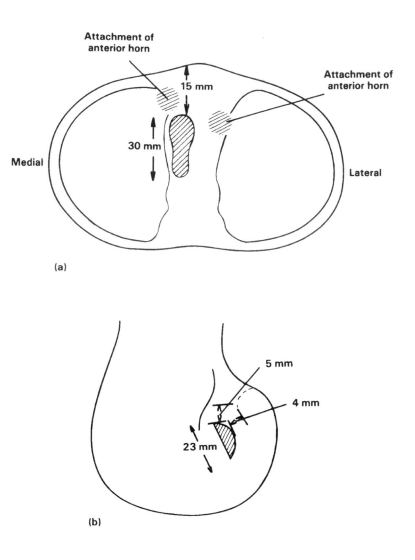

Figure 5.8 Placement of the substitute ligament can never be entirely isometric, but anatomical insertion should be mimicked as closely as possible. (a) The 'footprint' attachment of the anterior cruciate ligament to the proximal tibia viewed from above. (b) The equally broad attachment of the ligament to the medial surface of the lateral femoral condyle antero-inferior to the posterior femoral notch (right knee)

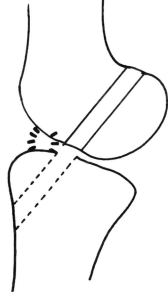

Figure 5.9 If the graft is placed too anteriorly, with the tibial tunnel anterior to the slope of the intercondylar roof, impingement during extension will lead to restricted movement and possible rupture of the graft

As yet there is no clear answer to the question about long-term benefits. Stability may be gained effectively in the short to medium term, with a return to sport at high level, but the eventual outcome is unknown compared to the natural history. It is to be hoped that clinical reviews in the next few years will address the issue, although comparative prospective, longitudinal studies are likely to be rare.

Alternatives to autografting

The interest in artificial ligaments has waned as longer term results reveal that rupture of the prosthesis is relatively common. Artificial fibres may be used as:

- A ligament in their own right (such as the Stryker Dacron polyester or ABC (composite of Dacron and carbon fibre yarns) prostheses)
- An augmentation device offering temporary support (Kennedy polypropylene LAD)

- A scaffold allowing a neoligament to form (Leeds Keio open weave polyester) (see Plate 49).

1 Availability
2 Ease of storage
3 No tissue loss
4 Quick operation
5 Early rehabilitation
6 Infection/contamination rare

Figure 5.10 *The advantages of a synthetic ligament*

The advantages of prosthetic replacement are obvious (Figure 5.10). The operation is relatively quick and the grafts are easy to handle, no morbidity from graft harvesting accrues and contamination is not a concern. Acceptable results at a mean of 3 years have been reported (Dahlstedt *et al.*, 1990; Macnicol *et al.*, 1991), although the presence of synovitis locally in relation to breakdown products and exposed polyester gives cause for concern (Figure 5.11; see also Plate 50). At present, synthetic ligaments should be restricted to further reconstruction or repeated revision for failed autogenous grafts, and perhaps as a primary procedure in the patient who is unlikely to place much demand upon the knee (Figure 5.12).

Allograft replacement offers many advantages if the graft can be harvested and stored safely. Ethylene oxide sterilization is now avoided since the ethylene glycol elicits a foreign body response, so contamination must be prevented, avoiding donors who have suffered viral infection such as hepatitis, AIDS, multiple sclerosis or Creutzfeld–Jacob disease. The Achilles, tibialis anterior, peroneal and toe flexor tendons are appropriate and should be stored at –70°C. Fresh frozen grafts are preferred to freeze-

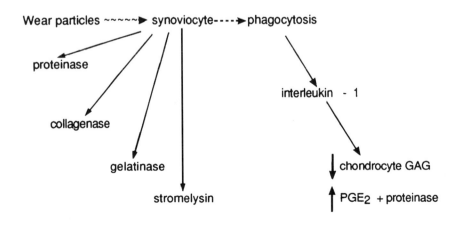

Figure 5.11 *Wear particles within the knee initiate an inflammatory response and the release of injurious enzymes*

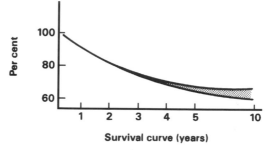

Figure 5.12 *The survival of a prosthesis depends upon its placement. After an early period of rupture or attrition, longer term results appear to show that the knees in the remainder of patients remain satisfactory. Autogenous grafting improves upon this survival curve*

dried tissue which may be more antigenic. Secondary sterilization by gamma irradiation (25,000 Gy) is also recommended, but both this and freezing cause the allograft to stretch under load, perhaps to a greater degree than with autografts, although both types are subjected to the same biological process of necrosis, revascularization and remodelling (Cabaud *et al.*, 1980; Shino *et al.*, 1984).

Artificial ligaments, perhaps made of processed collagen, or allografts may achieve a more defined role in knee ligament surgery in the future. They are indicated when there is a lack of available autogenous tissue, particularly in revisions, and possibly in the older patient. Where harvesting a strip of patellar tendon appears unwise owing to patellofemoral pathology, or malalignment, then there may again be a relative indication to avoid autogenous grafting.

Additional extra-articular grafting

Noyes and Barber (1991) considered that a combined intra-articular and lateral iliotibial band extra-articular procedure produced better arthrometric and functional results in chronic anterior cruciate deficiency than an intra-articular procedure alone. This was using allografts, but with autografts the consensus is that the addition of an extra-articular reconstruction, even in chronic and marked laxity, confers no definite benefit (Larson, 1993). A biomechanical study in human cadavers confirmed this impression (Amis and Scammell, 1993) and there is a risk that associated posterolateral laxity may become symptomatic.

Extra-articular procedures alone tend to slacken unacceptably and there seems to be little difference clinically between proximal (MacIntosh and Darby, 1976) or distal (Ellison, 1979) substitutions (Carson, 1988). However, in patients with relatively low athletic demands the lateral sling may be sufficient and avoids the risks associated with intra-articular surgery. Symptoms from the unphysiological positioning of the lateral band are, however, common (O'Brien *et al.*, 1991) and may outweigh the stabilizing effect. Where chronic laxity is multidirectional, the procedure may also worsen the component of posterolateral laxity which may not be fully appreciated preoperatively.

The ligament augmentation device (LAD)

Roth *et al.* (1985) and Dahlstedt *et al.* (1990) reported that an augmentation device improved the results of intra-articular autogenous patellar tendon reconstruction. Experimental studies in animals have shown that the prosthesis, usually of polypropylene braid (3M, St. Paul, Minnesota), protects the graft during the first year when it is at its weakest. The presence of artificial material in the knee may excite a foreign body reaction, however, and removal of the LAD is advised in a proportion of cases. Recently, Noyes and Barber (1992) found no advantage to accrue from the LAD when used in a prospective study using bone–patellar tendon–bone allografts. An absorbable stent of PDS Kordel (Ethicon) gives similar early results to the Kennedy LAD when used to protect a semitendinosus autograft (Macnicol and Sheppard, 1995), and since PDS disappears from the knee over a six-month period it offers a safe means of anchoring the tendon graft. The use of non-absorbable augmentation devices has waned in the same way as artificial ligaments, owing to concerns about the presence of particulate debris within the joint over many years.

As the surgical approach to anterior cruciate ligament rupture continues to evolve with arthroscopically-aided operations and rapid rehabilitation, a conservative approach may be acceptable in fewer patients with chronic deficiency, although many will still not report for later orthopaedic treatment after proven acute rupture (Macnicol, 1992). It must be remembered that the complications associated with poorly conducted surgery are rarely documented in the literature and that the graft probably never achieves the mechanical strength, viscoelasticity and proprioception of the natural ligament. Concerns persist about:

- The placement of the tissue, which can never be entirely isometric
- The multi-axial disposition and broad attachment of the ACL, which are unlikely to be reproduced
- The extent of the notchplasty
- The correct tensioning of the graft (since over-tightening may impair biological adaptation (Yoshiya *et al.*, 1987))
- The speed of postoperative loading of the knee

Nevertheless, it is an exciting field of surgical practice and the clinical improvement after successful reconstruction encourages an optimistic approach.

POSTERIOR CRUCIATE LIGAMENT TEARS

Rupture of the posterior cruciate ligament (PCL) may occur in isolation or in combination with other components of the knee. In chronic laxity the arcuate complex will stretch and posterolateral laxity becomes more obvious, followed by eventual laxity of the medial restraints. The mechanisms of injury include:

- A blow to the front of the flexed knee which drives the proximal tibia backwards, a relatively common occurrence in road traffic accidents and football tackles (the foot is usually fixed)

- Forced flexion of the knee, particularly if a load is applied to the body from above or the foot is plantarflexed
- Hyperextension of the knee which, after tearing the anterior cruciate ligament, will disrupt the PCL
- Major angulatory, rotational or distraction forces which effectively produce dislocation of the joint

Trickey (1968) reported that the ligament was most commonly avulsed from the tibial attachment, and certainly this is both the most likely site of the injury in the child and adolescent, and the most amenable to repair. However, so many cases of PCL rupture are neither diagnosed nor fully investigated that the incidence of tears at different levels is not accurately known; Insall (1984) suggests that upper, middle and lower third tears or avulsions occur in equal frequency. The PCL is ruptured relatively infrequently in sports injuries, and is more likely in soccer or rugby players than in skiers (Jakob, 1992). Certainly ACL rupture is 5–10 times more common and constitutes a reason for surgical intervention much more regularly.

The tests for cruciate and posterolateral laxity have been presented (see page 32) and many other modifications have been described (Jakob, 1992). The problem relates to the extent of the subsequent surgery, if that is felt to be indicated.

After acute rupture the clinical tests of a posterior drawer sign, tibial drop back and posterior shift (active and passive) of the lateral plateau are usually evident. The signs may be hard to elicit (Hughston, 1988), possibly because the arcuate complex is intact, and popliteal tenderness is not always evident, particularly in cases of femoral avulsion. A haemarthrosis, and restricted and painful flexion should alert the examiner to the possibility of PCL injury which can be confirmed by MR scan or arthroscopy using the 70° telescope. The posterior and mid-portions of the PCL are readily visualized, particularly through a central portal, although synovitis and haemorrhage may obscure the view. A posterolateral portal affords good access to all but the femoral attachment of the ligament.

Surgical reattachment of the ligament is advisable for ruptures less than 4–6 weeks old, particularly tibial bone avulsions (Trickey, 1968, 1980). The ligament should heal well in its vascular, retrosynovial site, whether there is bone avulsion or not. With mid-substance tears, reconstruction with semitendinosus or a strip of patellar tendon should be considered if posterior laxity exceeds the contralateral knee by more than 10 mm in association with persistent symptoms. Partial tears of the PCL, with intact ligaments of Wrisberg and Humphry, may allow the knee to compensate by quadriceps tone, so that acute intervention is unwarranted.

Access to the femoral attachment is through an anteromedial or longitudinal anterior incision. By means of a special tibial guide and a front-to-back bone tunnel the posterior insertion can be reached. Equally, the tibial end can be reached through a popliteal incision, carefully reflecting one or other head of the gastrocnemius and incising the oblique popliteal ligament and capsule. Complex laxity, involving the posterolateral and posteromedial corners of the knee, may require repair of popliteus and the biceps tendon, since these retract, and reefing of the arcuate complex proximally (Trillat, 1978) and the posteromedial capsule distally. It is important to correct varus laxity as much as possible, and the knee should be splinted in extension to prevent tibial sag postoperatively.

Unfortunately bracing of the knee fails to control posterior subluxation, and when fixed splintage is discontinued at 3–6 weeks, laxity may rapidly recur. Ligament augmentation with artificial fibres is therefore recommended, although this does not guarantee protection of the graft and breakdown products may produce a local synovitis later. The use of a patellotibial Steinmann pin to prevent postoperative tibial dropback ('olecranization') is not recommended as it cannot be left safely *in situ* for long.

The late results of posterior cruciate reconstruction are relatively disappointing for acute mid-substance, complex and late-diagnosed tears. But the principle of early restoration of ligament integrity should not be forgotten, confirmed by the satisfactory results of early intervention (Clancy *et al.*, 1983). Degenerative changes correlate with the degree of laxity (Torg *et al.*, 1989), and in the athlete particularly, surgical intervention is warranted.

LATERAL LIGAMENT COMPLEX INJURIES

The lateral structures of the knee which work together to stabilize the joint include the fibular collateral ligament, fascia lata, the popliteus muscle and tendon, the biceps femoris muscle, the lateral head of gastrocnemius, and the arcuate ligament. If the structures are disrupted, it is usual for the common peroneal nerve to be injured as it will also be stretched, and unfortunately the recovery after this traction injury to the nerve is minimal. It is difficult to distinguish which of the various lateral structures are principally injured, but in addition to varus laxity the knee may hyperextend and externally rotate if the leg is held by the toe or heel with the patient lying supine (Figure 5.13; see also Chapter 2).

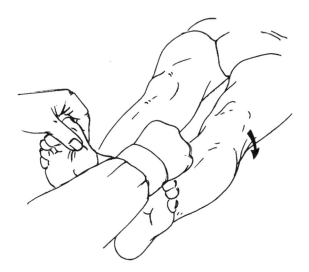

Figure 5.13 The genu recurvatum – external rotation test

This posterolateral instability can occur with an intact fascia lata, and the usual structures injured primarily are the fibular collateral ligament, the popliteus tendon and the arcuate complex. It is difficult clinically to distinguish posterolateral laxity from the hyperextension that occurs after the posterior cruciate ligament, and possibly the posterior capsule, have torn. If all posterior structures are ruptured, the medial tibial condyle, in addition to the lateral tibial condyle, subluxes posteriorly and radio-opaque markers on both medial and lateral sides of the joint may help to differentiate between posterior and posterolateral laxity.

Posterolateral laxity is best detected with the knee in 30° of flexion. If there is posterior subluxation of the tibia when the knee is 90° flexed, then the posterior cruciate ligament is probably also compromised. The reverse pivot shift test (Jakob *et al.*, 1981) is more likely to be positive than Hughston's external rotation recurvatum test (Hughston and Norwood, 1980), the posteriorly subluxed lateral tibial condyle reducing as the flexed knee is extended with the tibia externally rotated. Anterolateral and posterolateral laxity may coexist and are not necessarily symptomatic.

Treatment

Lateral ligament complex tears are symptomatic, the patient experiencing both instability and pain when standing. It is essential to repair the biceps tendon and the fascia lata as they will retract rapidly after injury. The fibular collateral ligament and the popliteus tendon attachment to the femoral condyle may be advanced anterosuperiorly, using a segment of bone incorporating their insertion to ensure an adequate reattachment. If the arcute ligament is well defined, this can be reefed additionally. Therefore, early repair is usually advisable and should secure a satisfactory result.

The complexities of surgical reconstruction for chronic posterolateral instability are beyond the scope of this book. Conservative management, emphasizing biceps and popliteus exercises, are more likely to succeed in the knee with valgus alignment. When the laxity coexists with varus, surgical reefing of the posterolateral structures (Trillat, 1978; Hughston and Jacobson, 1985) may have to be combined with a proximal tibial valgising osteotomy.

A ligament augmentation device or free autogenous graft may be necessary to bolster the reconstruction, and the extent of posterior cruciate insufficiency should be judged at surgery, although cruciate reconstruction is usually unnecessary.

References

Aglietti, P., Buzzi, R. and Zaccherotti, G. (1992) Patellar tendon versus semitendinosus and gracilis in ACL reconstruction. In *Meeting Abstracts and Outlines of the 18th Annual Meeting of the American Orthopaedic Society for Sports Medicine*, San Diego, pp. 29–30

Amis, A.A. and Scammell, B.E. (1993) Biomechanics of intra-articular and extra-articular reconstruction of the anterior cruciate ligament. *J. Bone Joint Surg.*, **75B**, 812–817

Annandale, T. (1885) An operation for displaced semilunar cartilage. *Br. Med. J.*, **1**, 779–781

Balkfors, B. (1982) The course of knee ligament injuries. *Acta Orthop. Scand.*, **198**, 1–91

Ballock, R.T., Woo, S. L.-Y., Lyon, R.M. *et al.* (1989) Use of patellar tendon autograft for anterior cruciate ligament reconstruction in the rabbit : a long-term histologic and biomechanical study. *J. Orth. Res.*, **7**, 474–485

Berchuck, M., Andriacchi, T.P., Bach, B.R. *et al.* (1990) Gait adaptations by patients who have a deficient anterior cruciate ligament. *J. Bone Joint Surg.*, **72A**, 8871–8877

Bonnet, A. (1845) *Traité des maladies des articulations*, Baillière, Paris

Cabaud, H.E., Feagin, J.A. and Rodkey, W.G. (1980) Acute anterior cruciate ligament injury and augmented repair. Experimental studies. *Am. J. Sports Med.*, **8**, 395–401

Cannon, W.D. Jr. and Vittori, J.M. (1992) The incidence of healing in arthroscopic meniscal repairs in anterior cruciate ligament-reconstructed knees versus stable knees. *Am. J. Sports Med.*, **20**, 176–181

Carson, W.G. (1988) The role of lateral extra-articular procedures for anterolateral rotatory instability. *Clin. Sports Med.*, **7**, 751–772

Clancy, W.G. Jr., Narechamia, R.G., Rosenberg, T.D. *et al.* (1981) Anterior and posterior cruciate ligament reconstruction in Rhesus monkeys : a histological, micro-angiographic and biomechanical analysis. *J. Bone Joint Surg.*, **63A**, 1270–1284

Clancy, W.G. Jr., Shelbourne, K.D., Zoellner, G.B. *et al.* (1983) Treatment of the knee joint instability secondary to rupture of the posterior cruciate ligament : report of a new procedure. *J. Bone Joint Surg.*, **65A**, 310–322

Dahlstedt, L., Dalen, N. and Jonsson, V. (1990) Gore-tex prosthetic ligament versus Kennedy ligament augmentation device in anterior cruciate ligament reconstruction : a prospective randomised 3-year follow-up of 41 cases. *Acta Orthop. Scand.*, **61**, 217–224

Daniel, D.M. (1990) Principles of knee ligament surgery. In *Knee Ligaments: Structure, Function, Injury and Repair* (eds Daniel, D.M., Akeson, W.H. and O'Connor, J.J.), Raven Press, New York, pp. 11–29

Ellison, A.E. (1979) Distal iliotibial-band transfer for anterolateral rotatory instability of the knee. *J. Bone Joint Surg.*, **61A**, 330–337

Engebretsen, L., Benum, P., Fasting, O. *et al.* (1990) A prospective randomised study of three surgical techniques for treatment of acute ruptures of the anterior cruciate ligament. *Am. J. Sports Med.*, **18**, 585–590

Hey-Groves, E.W. (1917) Operation for repair of the crucial ligaments. *Lancet*, **2**, 674–678

Holden, J.P., Grood, E.S., Butler, D.L. *et al.* (1988) Biomechanics of fascia lata ligament replacements : early post-operative changes in the goat. *J. Orth. Res.*, **6**, 639–647

Howell, S.M. and Taylor, M.A. (1993) Failure of reconstruction of the anterior cruciate ligament due to impingement by the intercondylar roof. *J. Bone Joint Surg.*, **75A**, 1044–1055

Hughston, J.C. (1988) The absent posterior drawer test in some acute posterior cruciate ligament tears of the knee. *Am. J. Sports Med.*, **16**, 39–43

Hughston, J.C. and Barrett, G.R. (1983) Acute anteromedial rotatory instability : long-term results of surgical repair. *J. Bone Joint Surg.*, **65A**, 145–153

Hughston, J.C. and Jacobson, K.E. (1985) Chronic posterolateral rotatory instability of the knee. *J. Bone Joint Surg.*, **67A**, 351–359

Hughston, J.C. and Norwood, L.A. Jr. (1980) The posterolateral drawer test and external rotation recurvatum test for posterolateral rotatory instability of the knee. *Clin. Orthop.*, **147**, 82–87

Indelicato, P.A. (1983) Non-operative treatment of complete tears of the medial collateral ligament of the knee. *J. Bone Joint Surg* **65A**, 323–329

Insall, J.N. (1984) Chronic instability of the knee. In *Surgery of the Knee* (ed Insall, J.N.), Churchill Livingstone, New York

Jakob, R.P. (1992) Acute posterior cruciate ligament tears – diagnosis and management. In *Knee Surgery : Current Practice* (eds Aichroth, P.M. and Cannon, D.W. Jr.), Martin Dunitz, London, pp. 322–328

Jakob, R.P., Hassler, H. and Stäubli, H.-U. (1981) Observations on rotatory instability of the lateral compartment of the knee : experimental studies on the functional anatomy and the pathomechanism of the true and reversed pivot shift sign. *Acta Orthop. Scand.*, **52** (Suppl. 191), 1–32

Johnson, R.J., Eriksson, E., Haggmark, T. *et al.* (1984) Five- to ten-year follow-up evaluation after reconstruction of the anterior cruciate ligament. *Clin. Orthop. Rel. Res.*, **183**, 122–140

Jonsson, T., Petersen, L. and Renström, P. (1990) Anterior cruciate ligament repair with and without augmentation : a prospective 7-year study of 51 patients. *Acta Orth. Scand.*, **61**, 562–566

Larson, R.L. (1993) Principles of replacement and reinforcement. In Mini Symposium: Knee Ligament Injuries. *Curr. Orthop.*, **7**, 94–100

MacIntosh, D.L. and Darby, T.A. (1976) Lateral substitution reconstruction. *J. Bone Joint Surg.*, **58B**, 142

Macnicol, M.F. (1989) The torn anterior cruciate ligament. *J. R. Coll. Surg. Edin.* **34** (Suppl.), 4–11

Macnicol, M.F. (1992) The conservative management of the anterior cruciate ligament-deficient knee. In *Knee Surgery, Current Practice* (eds Aichroth, P.M. and Cannon, W.D.), Martin Dunnitz, London, pp. 217–221

Macnicol, M.F., Penny, I.D. and Sheppard, L. (1991) Early results of Leeds–Keio anterior cruciate ligament replacement. *J. Bone Joint Surg.*, **73B**, 377–380

Macnicol, M.F. and Sheppard, L. (1995) A randomised, prospective trial of the Kennedy LAD versus a PDS Kordel stent in anterior cruciate ligament autogenous reconstruction. *J. Bone Joint Surg.* (in press)

Marder, R.A., Raskind, J.R. and Carroll, M. (1991) Prospective evaluation of arthroscopically assisted reconstruction. Patellar tendon vs semitendinosus and gracilis. *Am. J. Sports Med.*, **19**, 478–484

Noyes, F.R. and Barber, S.D. (1991) The effect of an extra-articular procedure on allograft reconstructions for chronic ruptures of the anterior cruciate ligament. *J. Bone Joint Surg.*, **73A**, 822–892

Noyes, F.R. and Barber, D.S. (1992) The effect of a ligament-augmentation device on allograft reconstruction for chronic ruptures of the anterior cruciate ligament. *J. Bone Joint Surg.*, **74A**, 960–973

Noyes, F.R., Delucas, J.L. and Torvik, P.J. (1974) Biomechanics of anterior cruciate ligament failure : an analysis of strain-rate sensitivity and mechanisms in primates. *J. Bone Joint Surg.*, **56A**, 236–253

O'Brien, S.J., Warren, R.F., Wickiewicz, T.L. *et al.* (1991) The iliotibial band lateral sling procedure and its effect on the results of anterior cruciate ligament reconstruction. *Am. J. Sports Med.*, **19**, 21–25

Palmer, I. (1938) On the injuries to the ligaments of the knee joint. A clinical study. *Acta Chir. Scand.*, **81**, Suppl. 53

Panni, A.S., Denti, M., Franzese, S. and Montaleone, M. (1993) The bone–ligament junction : a comparison between biological and artificial ACL reconstruction. *Knee Surg. Sports Traumatol. Arthroscopy*, **1**, 9–12

Pässler, H.H. (1993) The history of the cruciate ligaments : some forgotten (or unknown) facts from Europe. *Knee Surg. Sports Traumatol. Arthroscopy*, **1**, 13–16

Perry, J., Fox, J.M., Boitano, M.A. *et al.* (1980) Functional evaluation of the pes anserinus transfer by electromyography and gait analysis. *J. Bone Joint Surg.*, **62A**, 973–980

Roth, J.H., Kennedy, J.C., Lockstadt, H. *et al.* (1985) Polypropylene braid augmented and non-augmented intra-articular anterior cruciate ligament reconstruction. *Am. J. Sports Med.*, **13**, 321–336

Sachs, R.A., Daniel, D.M., Stone, M.L. and Garfein, R.F. (1989) Patellofemoral problems after anterior cruciate ligament reconstruction. *Am. J. Sports Med.*, **17**, 760–765

Sandberg, R., Balkfors, B., Nilsson, B. *et al.* (1987) Operative versus non-operative treatment of recent injuries to the ligaments of the knee. *J. Bone Joint Surg.*, **69A**, 1120–1126

Sgaghone, N.A., Del Pizzo, W., Fox, J.M. *et al.* (1993) Arthroscopic-assisted anterior cruciate ligament reconstruction with the pes anserine tendons : comparison of results in acute and chronic ligament deficiency. *Am. J. Sports Med.*, **21**, 249–256

Shelbourne, K.D. and Basle, J.R. (1988) Treatment of combined anterior cruciate ligament and medial collateral ligament injuries. *Am. J. Knee Surg.*, **1**, 56–58

Shelbourne, K.D., Wilekens, J.H., Mollabashy, A. and Decarlo, M. (1991) Arthrofibrosis in acute cruciate ligament reconstruction. The effect of timing on reconstruction and rehabilitation. *Am. J. Sports Med.*, **19**, 332–336

Shino, K., Kawasaki, T., Hirose, H., Gotoh, I. *et al.* (1984) Replacement of the anterior cruciate ligament by an allogenic tendon graft. An experimental study in the dog. *J. Bone Joint Surg.*, **66B**, 672–681

Smillie, I.S. (1978) *Injuries of the Knee Joint*, 5th edn, Churchill Livingstone, Edinburgh

Stark, J. (1850) Two cases of rupture of the crucial ligaments of the knee joint. *Edin. Med. Surg.*, **74**, 267–271

Torg, J.S., Barton, T.M., Pavlov, H. *et al.* (1989) Natural history of the posterior cruciate-deficient knee. *Clin. Orthop.*, **246**, 208–216

Trickey, E.L. (1968) Rupture of the posterior cruciate ligament of the knee. *J. Bone Joint Surg.*, **50B**, 334–341

Trickey, E.L. (1980) Injuries to the posterior cruciate ligament : diagnosis and treatment of early injuries and reconstruction of late instability. *Clin. Orthop. Rel. Res.*, **147**, 76–81

Trillat, A. (1978) Posterolateral instability. In *Late Reconstruction of Injured Ligaments of the Knee* (eds Schulitz, K.P., Krahl, H. and Stein, W.H.) Springer-Verlag, Berlin, pp. 99–105

Yoshiya, S., Andrish, J.T., Manley, M.T. *et al.* (1987) Graft tension in anterior cruciate ligament reconstruction. *Am. J. Sports Med.*, **15**, 464–470

6

Meniscal lesions

FUNCTION – STRUCTURES – HISTOLOGY – CLASSIFICATION
OF TEARS – MENISCECTOMY – JOINT LUBRICATION

FUNCTION

The role of the menisci of the knee is still debated, and it seems fruitless to list the different functions that have been suggested in any order of importance. The meniscus exerts a valuable and measurable effect upon the capabilities and resilience of the knee joint, and its total removal hastens degenerative changes in the affected compartment. The menisci contribute to the following functions:

- Distribution of load (approximately 55% through the lateral meniscus and 45% through the medial meniscus when the knee is straight)
- Improvement of congruency
- Enhancement of stability
- Nutrition of articular cartilage
- Lubrication

The first three actions are clearly interrelated, since the 'space-filler' effect of the menisci upon the tibial condyles ensures an efficient transmission of stress through the joint, including their role as part of the guiding mechanism during rotatory movements.

Throughout flexion and extension the menisci move with the tibia, to which they are attached, but in rotation they are more influenced by the movement of the femoral condyles. Thus, during knee movements the tibia is able to pursue a winding or helicoid course across the distal end of the femur, rotating externally in extension (the converse of the internally-directed 'screw home' action of the femur on the tibia), and internally on full flexion (Walker and Erkman, 1975).

This precise tracking of the two bones upon each other is therefore determined collectively by the shape of the articulating condyles, the menisci, and the cruciate ligaments which act as guide-ropes. If the normal, accommodative rotation is prevented then the menisci may become trapped within the joint, resulting either in tears within the substance of the meniscus, or peripheral detachments. Both stretching and crushing forces are involved (Figure 6.1), although significant external force is not a characteristic in the majority of cases.

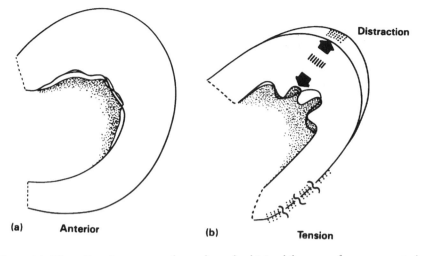

Posterior

Distraction

(a) **Anterior** **(b)** **Tension**

Figure 6.1 *Minor distortion occurs under moderate load (a), while greater force causes anterior horn tension and distraction of the posterior half of the meniscus (b)*

STRUCTURES

The anatomical and some of the functional differences of the two menisci are readily recognized. Although both structures are crescent shaped when viewed from above, the lateral meniscus is more nearly a complete circle. The anterior horns are anchored to the non-articular region of the tibia, in front of the anterior cruciate ligament insertion on the intercondylar eminence. Both anterior horns are linked by the transverse ligament which gives off bands of connective tissue that blend with the anterior cruciate ligament. The posterior horns are also attached to the intercondylar region of the tibia, but laterally there are additional anchorages since the lateral meniscus is moored to the medial femoral condyle in front of and behind the posterior cruciate ligament by the ligaments of Humphry and Wrisberg, respectively (the anterior and posterior meniscofemoral ligaments) (Figure 6.2). A similar fibrous band may also link the medial meniscus to the posterior cruciate ligament.

In cross-section the menisci are triangular, and viewed from behind the medial meniscus is narrower in front and broader posteriorly. The lateral meniscus is wider anteriorly than the medial meniscus and its width is more uniform, with a thicker outer margin. The peripheral attachments differ, since the medial meniscus is intimately blended with the capsule and the medial ligament, whereas the lateral meniscus is separated from the capsule posteriorly by the lateral ligament and the popliteus tendon. Hence the posterior half of the lateral meniscus is relatively free and can be drawn backwards by the popliteus muscle during internal rotation of the tibia upon the femur (Figure 6.3).

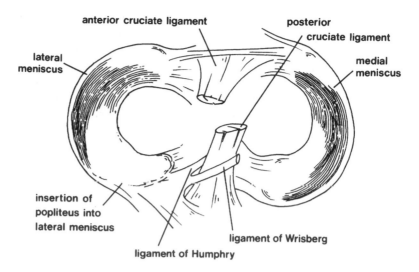

Figure 6.2 *Anatomy of the structures attached to the upper tibial surface, from in front: the anterior horn of the medial meniscus, the anterior cruciate ligament, the anterior and posterior horns of the lateral meniscus, the posterior horn of the medial meniscus, and the posterior cruciate ligament*

HISTOLOGY

Histological examination reveals that the menisci are predominantly collagenous, with a small amount of elastic tissue interspersed amid the connective tissue. They are therefore identifiably part of the ligamentous structure of the knee both medially and laterally. The fibres run circumferentially, resisting the bursting forces of weightbearing (Bullough *et al.*,

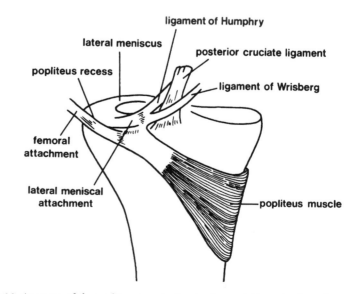

Figure 6.3 *Anatomy of the popliteus muscle showing its partial insertion into the posterior horn of the lateral meniscus*

1970), and are crossed, particularly in the central portion of the meniscus, by radial fibres (Figure 6.4). Nerves and blood vessels penetrate only the outer third and horns of the menisci, the remainder of the meniscus relying upon synovial fluid and diffusion for nutrition. Some collagen fibres accompanying the blood vessels in the periphery proceed radially through the circumferential fibres and form the inner edge of the meniscus. As these fibres are laminar rather than interwoven, they can be separated easily in the horizontal plane.

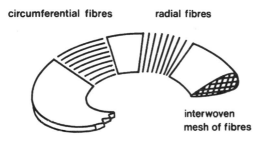

Figure 6.4 Histological structure of the meniscus showing the orientation of its collagen fibres

The innervation of the meniscus is shown in Figure 6.5. Mechanoreceptors are concentrated in the anterior and posterior horns, with a lesser distribution around the peripheral edge. Unmyelinated free nerve endings arborize as far as the middle third. Electron microscopy reveals that lymph channels extend throughout the full width of the meniscus and injection techniques define a network which may be absorptive, aiding in the nutrition of articular cartilage and meniscus.

Regeneration of a totally excised meniscus occurs by the centripetal growth of vascular fibrous tissue from the periphery of the joint. Possibly the initial haematoma is moulded into a wedge by the femoral condyle moving upon the tibia, and this then becomes organized by the ingrowth

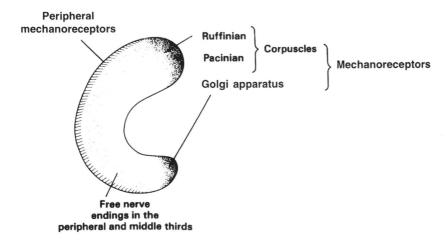

Figure 6.5 Innervation of the meniscus. Mechanoreceptors are congregated principally at both horns and along the peripheral margins

of connective tissue. This process cannot occur after a partial meniscectomy since the free edge of the meniscal remnant is not vascular. The regenerated meniscus is thinner and its inner margin is more rounded. The fibrous tissue is arranged irregularly and there is no obvious plane of cleavage peripherally as is seen in the normal meniscus.

CLASSIFICATION OF TEARS

Traumatic lesions of the meniscus generally occur vertically if they are produced acutely (see Figure 1.10). The classic mechanism of injury comprises a rotational stress upon the semi-flexed and weightbearing knee. A valgus or varus component may also be recalled, particularly if the leg has been involved in a collision, or if ligament laxity is present. Males are more commonly affected and there are said to be racial differences. Horizontal cleavage lesions are produced more insidiously and are usually associated with chronic stresses to the meniscus in a knee that is already slightly osteoarthritic.

Various types of meniscal tear are encountered (Figure 6.6), although different kinds, and sites, of tear frequently coexist. Trillat (1962) described the classic progression of a 'bucket handle' tear, commencing in the posterior third where arthroscopic access is most awkward. His anatomical classification was modified by Dandy (1990), but every surgeon with a large arthroscopic practice will have a slightly different impression of the pathological processes and their frequency. The components of the meniscal tears are:

Vertical: longitudinal – incomplete
                          bucket handle
                          pedunculated tag
            radial
            combined (flap)
Horizontal: posterior
            central
            anterior
            inner edge ('fishmouth') (see Figure 6.6)
            'parrot beak'
Complex: multiple vertical tears
            associated cystic changes (see Plate 43) (peripheral or central)

Cysts may also be encountered, affecting normal, congenitally abnormal and degenerative menisci. Figure 6.7 details the author's audit of 1350 tears encountered over a 5-year period.

Symptoms

Meniscal tears will produce pain, loss of movement and instability of the joint, and the interrelationship of these symptoms should be recognized. Pain arises from the stretching of the peripheral, sensory portion of the meniscus, and from the capsule and ligaments during the abnormal

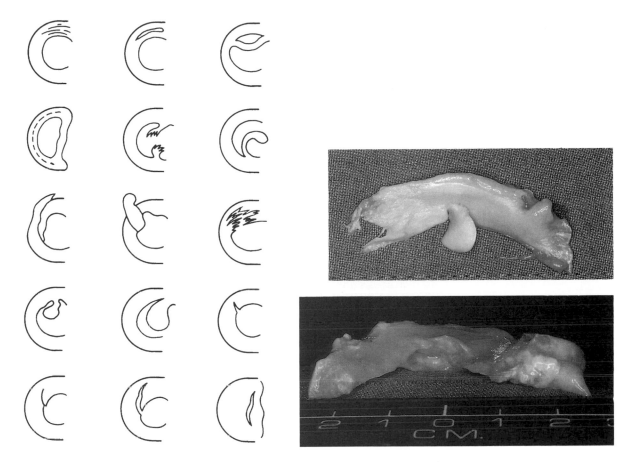

Figure 6.6 *Patterns of traumatic meniscal tears. The upper six diagrams show how a vertical tear may progress; various forms of tear are shown, in most of which the peripheral half of the meniscus can be preserved. A flap tear and a fishmouth lesion are shown to the right*

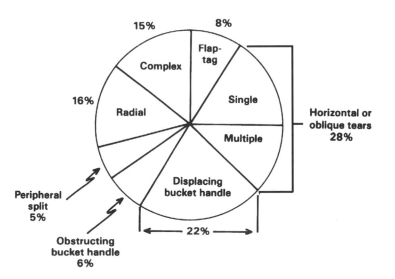

Figure 6.7 *Incidence of meniscal tears (as a percentage of a consecutive total of 1350)*

movement of the knee when an intra-articular obstruction is present. The body of the meniscus itself is insensitive.

Pain

Pain may be accompanied by clicking, or even a clunking sensation if the meniscus is displacing during flexion and extension. A limp may develop as the patient attempts to relieve the symptoms, and this limp may worsen towards the end of the day as the leg tires. Pain over the medial joint line, with tenderness when the knees touch together, is frequently complained of if the patient is asked about this directly; this feature is noticed in bed at night, but is not, as is classically taught, solely caused by a horizontal cleavage lesion.

Effusion

An effusion may be painful if it is tense, but this is unusual following a tear of the meniscus. If the knee becomes very swollen, and rapidly so, then a haemarthrosis should be suspected. As the meniscus is relatively avascular, a tear of a ligament and possibly also of the capsule should be suspected. Meniscal tears produce a lesser degree of swelling, the effusion gradually forming over the 12–24 hours after the injury. Thereafter, the fluid tends to disappear, but recurs when the joint is twisted or stressed subsequently.

Abnormal function

Mechanical problems are manifest by a sense of restricted extension and flexion, a feeling of stiffness, and a tendency for the joint to give way. In early tears, where the surface of the meniscus is little altered, the loss of joint movement may be very subtle, or absent. Stiffness will tend to lessen as the knee is exercised, and hence is at its worst early in the morning or after rest. Instability, or buckling, results not only from the obstruction in the joint altering the normal pivot, but also from muscle weakness or quadriceps inhibition. The patient complains that the joint is weak, or does not feel 'true', and a catching sensation occurs when the patient kneels, squats or jumps.

Signs

A torn meniscus produces joint line tenderness, often very localized, an effusion, which may be localized, as well as the more common total intrasynovial swelling and locking. The last term describes not simply a loss of full extension, but also restriction of flexion and rotation. The loss of extension is rarely more than 10–20°, and a greater loss suggests some other pathological lesion. In approximately 70% of cases these are the three cardinal signs of a torn meniscus.

However there may be quadriceps wasting in more chronic injuries, and a protrusion or localized area of oedema may be felt at the joint line. Ligaments may become tender and progressively lax owing to the abnormal mechanics of flexion, and patellofemoral pain and tenderness develop if the patient walks on a persistently flexed knee. Tenderness sometimes spreads over the femoral and tibial condyles, and the clinical picture thereby becomes confusing.

The McMurray test describes the production of a clunk or snapping sensation when the tibia is rotated with the knee in full flexion (McMurray, 1928). The test may be positive if a vertical, longitudinal tear is present in the posterior segment of the meniscus, and the fingers of one hand should palpate the joint line in order to improve precision. A somewhat similar grinding test has been described by Apley, whereby axial pressure is directed along the tibia which is again rotated, this time with the patient prone and the knee flexed at a right angle.

These tests for meniscal pathology are open to misinterpretation but are sometimes confirmatory. Eliciting pain by these manoeuvres is not pathognomonic of a meniscal tear, but the production of a clunk or abnormal movement may cause the patient to remark that the symptoms of instability have been reproduced. It is always as well to check that a similar clunk cannot be elicited in the opposite knee and examination of the knee on different occasions is recommended, particularly if the assessments are separated by a few weeks. There is certainly nothing to suggest that such delay will adversely influence the eventual outcome.

With the advent of readily available arthroscopic examination and MR scanning (see Chapter 3), early diagnosis and treatment of meniscal tears is possible, but is limited by health care restrictions and the availability of arthroscopically-trained surgeons.

MENISCECTOMY

Partial or total

The realization that the meniscus has a valuable function within the knee, even if only the peripheral portion is present, has led to a more conservative surgical policy when dealing with a tear (Figure 6.8) (Noble and Erat,

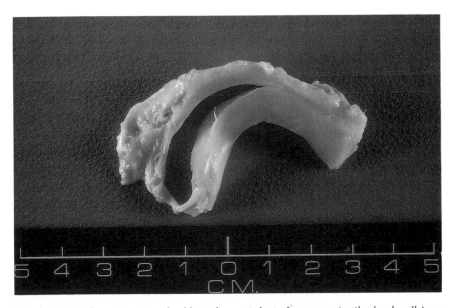

Figure 6.8 *Total meniscectomy should not be carried out for a posterior 'bucket handle' tear amenable to repair*

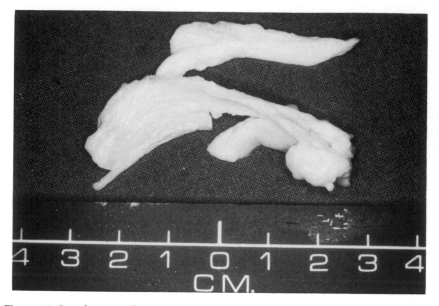

Figure 6.9 *Complex tears of a medial meniscus where excision was the only realistic surgical approach*

1980). The principal argument for removing the whole meniscus at operation was centred on the realistic concern that a further tear might otherwise be harboured within the remnant (Figure 6.9) and that regeneration of a pseudomeniscus was likely. Furthermore, an unstable residual rim of meniscus could, and indeed can, be the source of continuing pain and instability. Equally, the peripheral remnant of meniscus is important as it not only constitutes part of the capsular and ligamentous complex, but is also capable of transmitting a significant proportion of load. Hence its preservation is preferable.

Total meniscectomy in children is also known to give poor results (Fairbank, 1937; Zaman and Leonard, 1978) and the advent of arthroscopic surgery (Watanabe and Takeda, 1958), coupled with restricted meniscectomy (Suman *et al.*, 1984) or meniscal repair has reduced the morbidity of the procedure appreciably. Jones *et al.* (1978) also confirmed the disappointing results of meniscectomy in the older patient, where arthritic changes make for a less certain satisfactory outcome.

Comparisons of the results following partial, instead of total, meniscectomy confirm the benefits of conservative surgery (McGinty *et al.*, 1977; Dandy *et al.*, 1983), confining the excision to unstable or severely distorted meniscal tissue (Figure 6.10). The details of arthroscopic technique cannot be learnt from a book such as this. Access and triangulation skills remain the pivotal factors in achieving successful surgical excision or repair, and the methodology is clearly described in surgical atlases (Dandy, 1981; Johnson, 1986).

There is also some debate about whether a posterior horn remnant, not uncommonly left behind if the meniscus ruptures in its central portion during attempted removal, should be dissected out *in toto* through the potentially injurious posteromedial approach. Such retained segments are

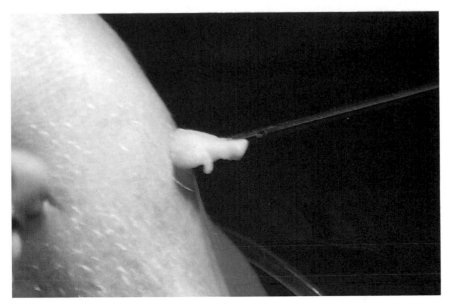

Figure 6.10 *Percutaneous removal of an excised, distorted 'bucket handle' through a medial portal*

probably better left initially, since a sizeable proportion of these cases will not become symptomatic after surgery. It is useful to re-arthroscope the knee before finally deciding to operate again as the residual meniscus may be fairly smooth and non-obstructive. Even after removal of a retained portion of meniscus, post-meniscectomy symptoms may persist (Table 6.1).

Table 6.1 Grading of results following meniscectomy*

Grading of result	Criteria
Excellent	No symptoms, no loss of movement, no effusions
Good	Minor symptoms after vigorous activity, no loss of movement, occasional effusion
Fair	Symptoms prevent vigorous activity, slight loss of flexion, occasional effusion
Poor	Symptoms interfere with everyday activities, loss of flexion and extension, regular effusions

*Symptoms are more persistent if the knee is unstable or arthritic.
From Tapper and Hoover (1969).

Prognosis after meniscectomy

The prognosis after meniscectomy is adversely affected by the following factors:

- Presence of osteoarthritis
- Presence of significant ligament laxity or other injuries

- Other meniscus already removed
- Young patient (poor results common in the child)
- Female sex

While the removal of part rather than all the meniscus is now widely practised, the skills required to perform 'arthroscopic meniscectomy' can only be achieved with careful training. As the current group of orthopaedic surgeons in training familiarize themselves with this demanding technique, a new generation of arthroscopists increasingly practises this surgical skill as a specialty in its own right.

Complications following arthroscopic procedures are detailed in Table 3.5. The articular cartilage may be scuffed and lacerated by careless use of the instruments, and there is the risk that inadequate excision of abnormal tissue may occur in inexperienced hands. Nevertheless, convalescence after arthroscopic meniscectomy is certainly faster, characterized by day-case surgery and a speedier return to work and sport.

Osteoarthritic changes are hastened by meniscectomy, and are more obvious after total meniscectomy (Parry *et al.*, 1958). Indeed, it is now known that following a meniscectomy approximately one-third of patients will suffer from the clinical and radiographic signs of osteoarthritis, and a meniscectomy in childhood introduces a 70% risk of significant degenerative changes after 20 years (Suman *et al.*, 1984). Degeneration of the articular cartilage not only occurs where it is exposed after surgery, but also appears below a regenerated, but false, meniscus.

If a tear in the meniscus continues to block normal knee function, then this too will bring about an arthritic process; yet there is little to suggest that the retention of an abnormal meniscus will lead to a greater deterioration in the knee than occurs after total meniscectomy, and the prevention of arthritis must never be used as a reason for meniscal excision. Rather, it should be the relief of pain and the improvement of function that act as indications for this form of surgery. Conceivably, ligament integrity is also preserved by the removal of an obstruction in the joint.

The radiographic features of osteoarthritis that follow meniscectomy (Figure 6.11) include:

- Ridge formation
- Generalized flattening of the marginal half of the femoral condyle
- Narrowing of the joint space
- Localized osteophyte formation

The signs are in no way specific and the incidence of this complication is therefore difficult to gauge. The osteoarthritis is progressive, and hence the incidence varies also with the length of follow-up.

Meniscal repair

The vascularity of the meniscus diminishes from its peripheral edge centrally. Healing will occur dependably in the outer third due to its proximity to the capsular attachment (Heatley, 1980; Arnoczky and Warren, 1982). The central third tear will coapt if held together accurately and there is evidence that fibrochondrocytes in the avascular zone can be

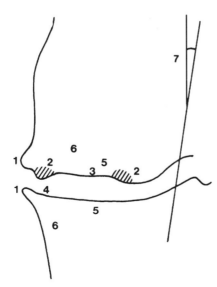

Figure 6.11 Post-meniscectomy radiographic changes. 1–osteophyte formation; 2–ridge formation; 3–generalized flattening of the marginal half of the femoral condyle; 4–narrowing of the joint space; 5–sclerosis of the subchondral plate on either side of the joint; 6–occasional cyst formation; 7–angulatory deformity of the knee

activated by blood components experimentally (Arnoczky *et al.*, 1988), although the use of a homologous fibrin clot or fibrin glue (Ishimura *et al.*, 1991) in clinical studies has not yet proved of value. A tear in the substance of the meniscus which extends peripherally may heal, as shown by King (1936) in his classic study in the dog, cellular ingrowth stemming from peripheral synovial and subsynovial cells. Henning *et al.* (1991) has pioneered the use of an autologous fascial sheath to cover the repaired meniscus and to retain exogenous fibrin clot. The technique is demanding and the risk of injury to the articular surfaces is high.

Repair of the meniscus was successfully achieved by Thomas Annandale of Edinburgh in 1885. He used chromic catgut sutures to retain a peripheral tear of the anterior horn of the medial meniscus in a miner from Newcastle (Annandale, 1885). Meniscal repair was popularized by DeHaven (1985), who published a 10-year experience. Cooper *et al.* (1991) have provided detailed studies of the technique. Channels produced by the sutures allow the ingrowth of cells, and the edges of the tear should be debrided. Successful healing is more likely in the stable knee and age does not appear to influence the outcome (Hamberg *et al.*, 1983). A peripheral split of the medial or lateral meniscus is commonly encountered with anterior cruciate ligament tears, so both the ligament and the meniscus can be dealt with concurrently. Grossly distorted and chronically displaced meniscal tears are unsuitable for suture.

Techniques of repair include the use of a double-barrel curved cannula system, inserting long needles linked by a 2–0 PDS suture from inside-out (Clancy and Graf, 1983), an outside-in method where knotted PDS sutures are pulled peripherally (Warren, 1985) and an inside-inside technique, suturing the meniscal portions together arthroscopically (Morgan *et al.*,

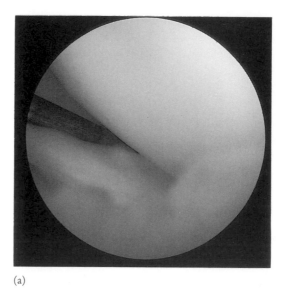

Figure 6.12(a,b) At arthroscopy a blunt hook confirms the presence of a displacing 'bucket handle' tear of the medial meniscus

(a)

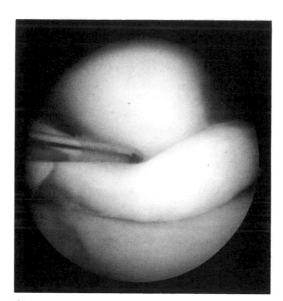

(b)

1991) (Figures 6.12a,b–6.14). With all these methods the incidence of cartilage damage and neurovascular complications may be too high a price to pay for the purported reduction in the risks of later osteoarthritis, (Small, 1988).

Meniscal transplantation

Garrett and Stevenson (1991) propose that transplantation of menisci will reduce the incidence of osteoarthritis after total meniscectomy and may also lessen instability in the anterior cruciate-deficient knee. Clinical experience with this technique is still limited to a few centres but undoubtedly further

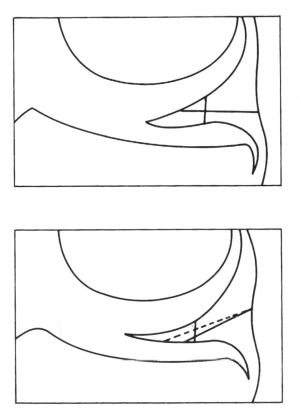

Figure 6.13 Sutures may be placed through the superior or inferior meniscal surface

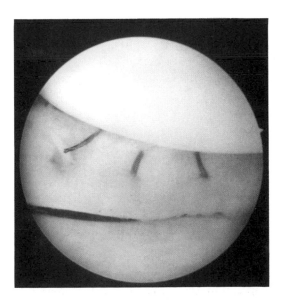

Figure 6.14 Meniscal sutures retaining the reduced 'bucket handle' segment

reports about the results will be forthcoming over the years. As with meniscal repair, an associated anterior cruciate ligament rupture should be recon-
structed since survival of the meniscus is otherwise endangered. Conversely,
knee stability may be achieved by combining meniscal transplantation with
anterior cruciate ligament surgery in cases where a total meniscectomy has
been carried out.

Since the provision of suitably sized and safe meniscal allografts may
prove to be a limiting factor in the future, experimental studies have
assessed Teflon net substitutes in the dog (Toyonoga *et al.*, 1983) and collagen implants may prove to be another way forward, both for meniscal
(Stone *et al.*, 1990) and ligament replacement.

The discoid lateral meniscus

The discoid meniscus probably forms as a result of its unusually mobile
attachments, since the abnormality is not seen in other animals (Kaplan,
1957). Classically the shapes have been divided into the complete, covering
the lateral tibial condyle, incomplete and highly mobile Wrisberg types
(Figure 6.15) (Watanabe *et al.*, 1979). Fujikawa *et al.* (1978) proposed that
a reduction in the lateral femoral condylar angle allowed the lateral meniscus to remain discoid (Figure 6.16) and described an anterior megahorn
meniscus which might develop if only the posterior half of the meniscus
was resorbed normally.

The discoid anomaly appears to be more common in the Chinese and
Japanese, but in the West the incidence is approximately 2.5% (Smillie,
1948). Symptoms include snapping (Middleton, 1936), pain, locking, limp,

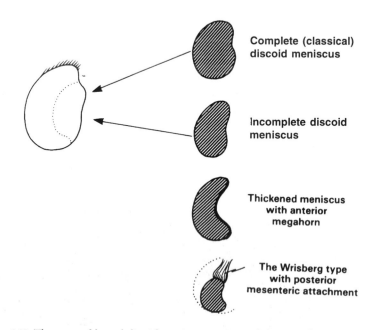

*Figure 6.15 The types of lateral discoid meniscus. Excision of the central portion of a classical
discoid meniscus may preserve its function (left), but the Wrisberg type usually merits complete
excision*

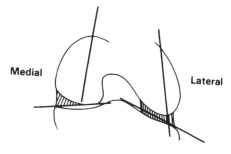

Medial   **Lateral**

Figure 6.16 Reduction in the lateral femoral condylar angle may predispose towards the formation of a discoid lateral meniscus (From Fujikawa et al., 1978)

effusions and giving way (Glasgow *et al.*, 1982). Aichroth *et al.* (1992) report that the classic clunk can only be elicited in 39% of knees and in some cases movement within the lateral compartment is seen or felt without a snap. The joint line may feel full and is often tender.

Other causes of snapping knee are patellofemoral instability, a subluxing iliotibial band, subluxation of the tibiofemoral or proximal tibiofibular joints and other meniscal pathology, particularly cystic change. The diagnosis can be established by arthroscopy which allows the morphology of the anomaly to be assessed, together with any tears involving the superior or inferior surfaces.

A conservative surgical approach is justifiable, so that medial edge tears should be saucerized and a partial, central meniscectomy carried out for more extensive lesions (Ikeuchi, 1982; Hayashi *et al.*, 1988). Excellent results have been reported in the short-term (Bellier *et al.*, 1989), although other reviews are less optimistic (Vandermeer and Cunningham, 1989). The troublesome Wrisberg type merits complete excision, as do discoid menisci

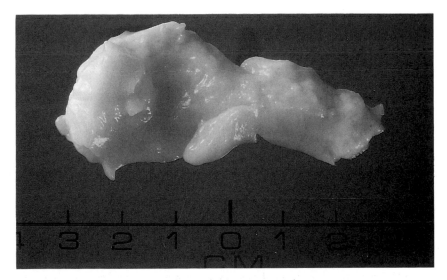

Figure 6.17 Multiple surface irregularities and a flap tear of an excised Wrisberg-type discoid meniscus

with major tears (Figure 6.17). In approximately 20% of cases the anomaly is bilateral, yet symptoms rarely affect both knees.

Complications of open meniscectomy

The immediate complications of meniscectomy by arthrotomy are:

- Haemarthrosis
- Wound infection
- Deep venous thrombosis
- Tourniquet paralysis
- Popliteal nerve palsy
- Damage to the popliteal vessels
- Capsular herniation
- Damage to the infrapatellar branch of the saphenous nerve
- Injury to other structures in the knee (Figure 6.18).

The late complications, apart from osteoarthritis, include recurrent effusions, knee stiffness, pain and a secondary malfunction of the patellofemoral joint.

Perhaps the worst complication of all is the removal of a normal meniscus, or one that is not the primary cause of symptoms. In the child, where locking and other internal derangements of the knee are increasingly frequent, with a male to female ratio of two to one, the accuracy of clinical diagnosis is less than 50%. Even in the adolescent, diagnostic accuracy from the history and physical examination does not exceed 66% and it is quite wrong to subject the knee to arthrotomy without prior arthroscopy. Confident clinical diagnosis of a medial meniscus vertical tear or a discoid lateral meniscus are all too commonly shown by arthroscopy to be erroneous. A convincingly locked knee may reveal no more than a minor synovial fringe lesion, fat-pad swelling or an early osteochondritic lesion when viewed with the

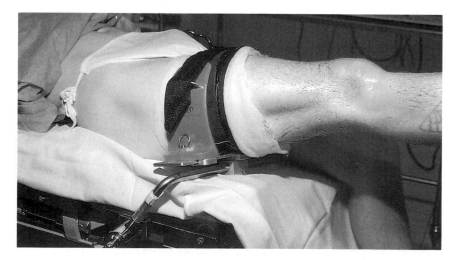

Figure 6.18 Excessive angulatory or rotational force when using the leg holder may produce ligamentous and capsular tears

arthroscope. It is better to err on the side of conservation in this age group, and also in those with degenerative changes in the knee.

JOINT LUBRICATION

The synovial membrane secretes a fluid which ensures that the coefficient of friction between the femur and the tibia, and the femur and the patella, is low. In articular joints the coefficient approaches 0.002 which compares very favourably with steel on ice (0.01). The coefficient of friction in artificial joints is in the region of 0.1.

Lubrication in the knee joint is of mixed type, with both fluid-film and boundary characteristics. In the fluid-film form, the apposing surfaces are separated by a thin film of fluid, many molecules thick. There are three forms of fluid-film lubrication:

- Hydrodynamic, which depends upon the motion of one surface upon the other
- Elastohydrodynamic, which includes a component of elastic deformation of one or both surfaces as a result of contact pressures
- 'Squeeze' film, where loading of the joint surfaces wrings out fluid from the articular cartilage and thus ensures preservation of the fluid-film even with considerable loading

The other form of lubrication is known as boundary lubrication, and here surface deformation occurs because a continuous fluid-film is not constantly present. It is known that gel-like substances aggregate on the surface of articular cartilage and this is proportional to the protein content of the synovial fluid.

In the knee joint, fluid-film and boundary lubrication exist together, although the fluid-film form is generally operant. When lubrication is insufficient, either as a result of injury or adverse metabolic processes, articular surfaces are subject to greater stresses, both compressive and frictional. Repeated haemarthroses, or the presence of debris and loose bodies, will also exert an adverse effect upon the properties of synovial fluid, and the increased wear within the joint will lead to osteoarthritis. It is apposite to conclude this chapter with the reminder that the menisci combine with the synovium and its secreted fluid to ensure that the articular cartilage of the knee joint is effectively lubricated and nourished.

References

Aichroth, P.M., Patel, D.V. and Marx, C.L. (1992) Congenital discoid lateral meniscus : a long-term follow-up study. In *Knee Surgery: Current Practice* (eds Aichroth, P.M. and Cannon, W.D.), Martin Dunitz, London, pp. 540–545

Annandale, T. (1885) An operation for displaced semilunar cartilage. *Br. Med. J.*, **1**, 779

Arnoczky, S.P. and Warren, R.F. (1982) Microvasculature of the human meniscus. *Am. J. Sports Med.*, **10**, 90–95

Arnoczky, S.P., Warren, R.F. and Spivak, J.M. (1988) Meniscal repair using an exogenous fibrin clot – an experimental study in dogs. *J. Bone Joint Surg.*, **70A**, 1209–1220

Bellier, G., Dupont, J.-Y., Larrain, M. *et al.* (1989) Lateral discoid menisci in children. *Arthroscopy*, **5**, 52–56

Bullough, P., Munera, L., Murphy, J. and Weinstein, A.M. (1970) The strength of the menisci as it relates to their fine structure. *J. Bone Joint Surg.*, **52B**, 64–70

Clancy, W.G. and Graf, B.K. (1983) Arthroscopic meniscal repair. *Orthopaedics*, **6**, 1125–1128

Cooper, D.E., Arnoczky, S.P. and Warren, R.F. (1991) Meniscal repair. *Clin. Sports Med.*, **10**, 529–548

Dandy, D.J. (1981) *Arthroscopic Surgery of the Knee*, Churchill Livingstone, Edinburgh

Dandy, D.J. (1990) Arthroscopic anatomy of symptomatic meniscal lesions. *J. Bone Joint Surg.*, **72B**, 628–631

Dandy, D.J., Northmore-Ball, M.D. and Jackson, R.W. (1983) Arthroscopie, open partial and total meniscectomy : a comparative study. *J. Bone Joint Surg.*, **65B**, 400–404

DeHaven, K.E. (1985) Meniscus repair in the athlete. *Clin. Orthop.*, **198**, 31–35

Fairbank, H.A.T. (1937) Internal derangement of the knee in children and adolescents. *Proc. R. Soc. Med.*, **30**, 427–432

Fujikawa, K., Tomatsu, T. and Malso, K. (1978) Morphological analysis of meniscus and articular cartilage in the knee joint by means of arthrogram. *J. Jpn Orthop. Ass.*, **52**, 203–215

Garrett, J.C. and Stevenson, R.N. (1991) Meniscal transplantation in the human knee: a preliminary report. *Arthroscopy*, **7**, 52–62

Glasgow, M.M.S., Aichroth, P.M. and Baird, P.R.E. (1982) The discoid lateral meniscus: a clinical review. *J. Bone Joint Surg.*, **64B**, 245–250

Hamberg, P., Gillquist, J. and Lysholm, J. (1983) Suture of new and old peripheral meniscus tears. *J. Bone Joint Surg.*, **65A**, 193–197

Hayashi, L.K., Yamaga, H., Ida, K. *et al.* (1988) Arthroscopic meniscectomy for discoid lateral meniscus in children. *J. Bone Joint Surg.*, **70A**, 1495–1500

Heatley, F.W. (1980) The meniscus – can it be repaired? *J. Bone Joint Surg.*, **62B**, 397–400

Henning, C.E., Yearout, M., Vequist, S.W. *et al.* (1991) Use of the fascia sheath coverage and exogenous fibrin clot in the treatment of complex meniscal tears. *Am. J. Sports Med.*, **19**, 626–631

Ikeuchi, H. (1982) Arthroscopic treatment of the discoid lateral meniscus : technique and long-term results. *Clin. Orthop.*, **167**, 19–28

Ishimura, M., Tamai, S. and Fujisawa, Y. (1991) Arthroscopic meniscal repair with fibrin glue. *Arthroscopy*, **7**, 177–181

Johnson, L.L. (1978) *Diagnostic and Surgical Arthroscopy*, 3rd edn, Mosby, St Louis

Jones, R.E., Smith, E.C. and Reisch, J.S. (1978) Effects of medial meniscectomy on patients older than forty years. *J. Bone Joint Surg.*, **60A**, 783–786

Kaplan, E.B. (1957) Discoid lateral meniscus of the knee joint. Nature, mechanism and operative treatment. *J. Bone Joint Surg.*, **39A**, 77–87

King, D. (1936) The healing of semilunar cartilages. *J. Bone Joint Surg.*, **18B**, 333–342

McGinty, J.B., Geuss, L.E. and Marvin, R.A. (1977) Partial or total meniscectomy. A comparative analysis. *J. Bone Joint Surg.*, **59A**, 763–766

McMurray, T.P. (1928) The diagnosis of internal derangements of the knee. In *Robert Jones Birthday Volume*, Oxford Medical Publications, Oxford, pp. 301–305

Middleton, D.S. (1936) Congenital disc-shaped lateral meniscus with snapping knee. *Br. J. Surg.*, **24**, 246–255

Morgan, C.D., Wojtys, E.M., Casscells, C.D. *et al.* (1991) Arthroscopic meniscal repair evaluated by second-look arthroscopy. *Am. J. Sports Med.*, **19**, 632–638

Noble, J. and Erat, K. (1980) In defence of the meniscus; a prospective study of two hundred meniscectomy patients. *J. Bone Joint Surg.*, **62B**, 6–11

Parry, C.B.W., Nichols, P.J.R. and Lewis, N.R. (1958) Meniscectomy: a review of 1,723 cases. *Ann. Phys. Med.*, **4**, 201–209

Small, N.C. (1988) Complications in arthroscopic surgery performed by experienced arthroscopists. *Arthroscopy*, **4**, 215–221

Smillie, I.S. (1948) The congenital discoid meniscus. *J. Bone Joint Surg.*, **30B**, 671–682

Stone, K.R., Rodkey, W.G., Webber, R.J. *et al* (1990) Future directions : collagen-based prostheses for meniscal regeneration. *Clin. Orthop.*, **252**, 129–135

Suman, R.K., Stother, I.G. and Illingworth, G. (1989) Diagnostic arthroscopy of the knee in children. *J. Bone Joint Surg.*, **66B**, 535–537

Tapper, E. and Hoover, N. (1969) Late results after meniscectomy. *J. Bone Joint Surg.*, **51A**, 517–526

Toyonaga, T., Vezaki, N. and Chikama, H. (1983) Substitute meniscus of teflon net for the knee joint of dogs. *Clin. Orthop.*, **179**, 291–297

Trillat, A. (1962) Lésions traumatique du ménisque interne du genu. Classement anatomique et diagnostic clinique. *Rev. Chir. Orthop.*, **48**, 551–563

Vandermeer, R.D. and Cunningham, F.K. (1989) Arthroscopic treatment of the discoid lateral meniscus : results of long-term follow-up. *Arthroscopy*, **5**, 101–109

Walker, P.S. and Erkman, M.H. (1975) The role of the menisci in force transmission across the knee. *Clin. Orthop.*, **104**, 184–193

Warren, R.F. (1985) Arthroscopic meniscus repair. *Arthroscopy*, **1**, 170–172

Watanabe, M. and Takeda, S. (1958) On the popularisation of arthroscopy. *J. Jpn Orthop. Ass.*, **27**, 258–261

Watanabe, M., Takeda, S. and Ikeuchi, H. (1979) *Atlas of Arthroscopy*, Igaku Shoin, Tokyo

Zaman, M. and Leonard, M.A. (1978) Meniscectomy in children : a study of fifty-nine knees. *J. Bone Joint Surg.*, **60B**, 436–437

7
Patellofemoral problems

CONGENITAL DISLOCATION – HABITUAL DISLOCATION –
RECURRENT SUBLUXATION AND DISLOCATION –
TREATMENT OF PATELLAR INSTABILITY – RETROPATELLAR
PAIN

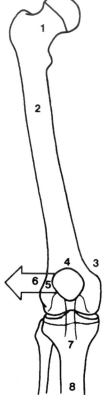

The injury which promotes patellar symptoms may clearly be recorded as a single event by the patient or may be cumulative. In many instances, no trauma can be recalled, the patellofemoral joint aching during periods of rapid growth in early adolescence or after repetitive use of the knee during certain occupations or in athletics.

Although it is important to differentiate between the group of patients whose patellae are dislocating or subluxing and those whose patellar tracking appears to be normal, the two groups are not easy to separate and there are undoubtedly a number of cases with subclinical (undetectable) subluxation of the patellofemoral joint. In certain instances the patella may tilt rather than sublux, and the term 'patellar instability' is to be preferred in these cases.

Yates and Grana (1990) use the term 'patellofemoral dysplasia' to describe a continuum of anatomical variations which predisposes the child to patellar symptoms. Many of these reside at sites distant from the patellofemoral joint (Figures 7.1 and 7.2a,b) combining torsional abnormalities with deficient connective tissue strength and morphological oddities of the joint itself. One important factor in most cases of dislocation during earlier childhood is relative shortening of the quadriceps mechanism. This is invariably present in the congenital forms of knee dislocation and subluxation (Figure 7.3), where recurvatum and restricted flexion are the norm.

Patellar dislocation is conveniently graded as:

(a) Congenital, in association with other gross anomalies noted at birth
(b) Habitual, coming to light in the first half of childhood
    (i)   during flexion
    (ii) during extension
    (iii) persistent, where the patella remains permanently out of the femoral groove
(c) Recurrent, often after relatively trivial injury
    (i)   acute onset with subsequent repeated episodes
    (ii) chronic, with gradual onset of instability

Figure 7.1 Sites where morphological abnormalities may predispose towards lateral patellar dislocation or subluxation (1, increased femoral neck anteversion; 2, internal (medial) femoral torsion; 3, weak vastus medialis muscle; 4, high or abnormally shaped patella; 5, deficient lateral femoral condyle; 6, tight lateral retinacular bands; 7, laterally-placed tibial tuberosity; 8, external tibial torsion)

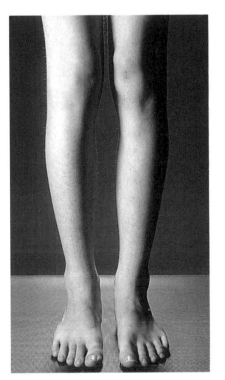

(a)

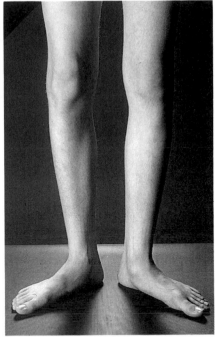

(b)

Figure 7.2 Persistent femoral anteversion producing inward squinting patellae (a) and compensatory external tibial torsion (b)

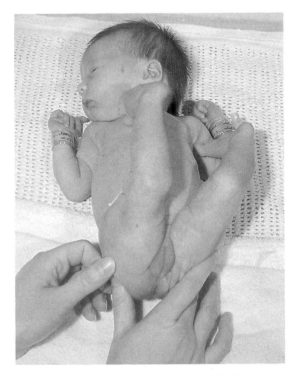

Figure 7.3 Congenital dislocation of the knee

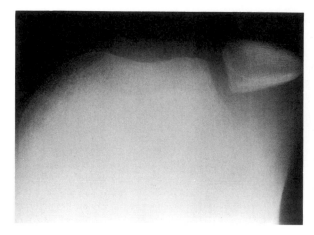

(a)

Figure 7.4 Lateral
patellar dislocation
viewed on (a) 'skyline'
and (b) oblique radio-
graphs

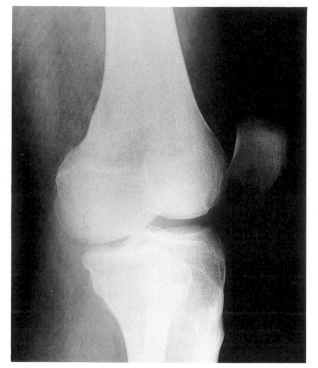

(b)

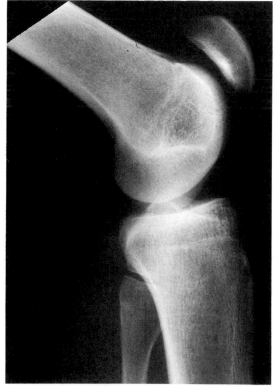

Figure 7.5 Patella alta

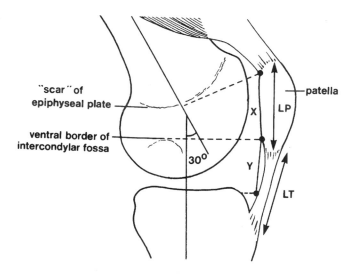

"scar" of
epiphyseal plate

ventral border of
intercondylar fossa

patella

LP

X

30°

Y

LT

Figure 7.6 Suggested measurements to describe patella alta. (1)
Blumensaat (1932) considered that the patella normally lies between
the dotted lines, which are extensions of the epiphysial line and the
intercondylar fossa with the knee in 30° of flexion. (2) Insall and
Salvati (1971) stated that LT : LP should not exceed 1.2; the distal end
of the patellar tendon, and hence the length of LT, is difficult to define
radiographically. (3) Blackburne and Peel (1977) used the ratio Y : X
since this uses the upper end of the tibia as a point of reference; normal
values are less than 1.0

Although dislocation is normally lateral (Figure 7.4a,b), inferior, superior (vertical) and medial displacement may also occur. Patella alta (Figures 7.5 and 7.6) and variations in the congruency angle of the patellofemoral joint have been defined radiographically (Merchant *et al.*, 1974) (Figure 7.7) and by CT scanning (Fulkerson *et al.*, 1987). These measurements are applicable clinically but do not fully reflect the complexity of patellar biomechanics.

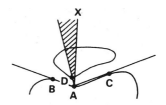

Figure 7.7 The sulcus (condylar groove or trochlear) angle BAC is constructed by the highest points of the medial (B) and lateral (C) condyles and the deepest part of the sulcus (A). The congruence angle XAD is the angle between the line bisecting the sulcus angle (AX) and the line linking the apex of the patella (D) and A. A congruence angle of over 5° suggests patellar subluxation (After Merchant et al., 1974)

CONGENITAL DISLOCATION

This condition is often associated with a skeletal dysplasia or motor retardation. The child is slow to walk or may be unable to weightbear effectively on the leg. In addition to the quadriceps contracture the femoral condylar groove is shallow with poor development of the lateral femoral condyle. The patella is usually oval and dysplastic, and its distal attachment may be laterally placed. Torsional deformity of the femur and tibia, soft-tissue laxity or contracture and foot abnormalities are common.

Since stretching and splintage of the knee in flexion usually fails when there is fixed deformity, treatment of the condition involves a lengthening of the rectus femoris and vastus lateralis, release of vastus intermedius and double breasting of the medial parapatellar structures, including vastus medialis (Goa *et al.*, 1990). Distal realignment of the patellar tendon should be achieved by rerouting its lateral half medially. Significant external tibial rotation is sometimes encountered and a concomitant pesplasty is then advisable. However, extensive realignment of musculotendinous units around the knee should not be undertaken lightly and it is often better to stage procedures, correcting the short quadriceps mechanism first and the torsional abnormalities in later childhood if patellar stability is not secured.

Following this extensive surgical release the knee is splinted in 20–30° of flexion for 6 weeks. The child is readmitted to hospital when the plaster is bivalved and physiotherapy is arranged as an inpatient. Full flexion is rarely restored, but a flexion arc of over 90° can usually be obtained. If the fascia lata remains relatively tight the Ober test (Ober, 1936) will be positive, demonstrated by the presence of an abductor contracture when the knee is extended.

HABITUAL DISLOCATION

In children where the quadriceps mechanism is relatively short, marked genu recurvatum will not be present but the patella will rest high in the femoral groove or above it. Coupled with this are other features of knee dysplasia, including a shallow femoral groove, axial and angulatory malalignment and ligament laxity. These are constitutional abnormalities, differentiating the problem from acquired quadriceps fibrosis following injections into the thigh during infancy (Gunn, 1964). Williams (1968) described patellar dislocation secondary to injections later in childhood, in contrast to restricted knee flexion without patellar dislocation in the infantile form of this iatrogenic condition.

Habitual dislocation may be familial and is seen in ligament laxity syndromes (Carter, 1960) and the hypermobility associated with the Ehlers–Danlos, Marfan's, Down's and Ellis–van Creveld syndromes, or other skeletal dysplasias such as onycho-osteodysplasia (nail-patella syndrome) and osteogenesis imperfecta. The onset of symptoms is gradual with no convincing trauma as a precipitant. Patella alta is usually obvious and the patella either shifts laterally under load during the last 20° of extension (Figure 7.8) or subluxes as the knee is flexed. In the latter variety an abnormal attachment of the iliotibial band into the lateral border of the patella may be palpable. In some children the patella tracks in a sinusoidal manner, moving out of the femoral sulcus in both extension and mid-flexion.

When these abnormalities of tracking become painful the child ceases to cope with sports, and even walking and sitting become troublesome. Physiotherapy may help in a proportion of cases, but persistence of the symptoms is common and disabling. Lateral release alone is ineffectual unless the dislocation occurs in flexion and a lateral tether can be demonstrated. If the quadriceps mechanism is short, a V–Y or Z lengthening is indicated, combined with a Goldthwaite–Roux medialization of the patellar tendon. The leg is splinted in a cast postoperatively, and after 6 weeks a period of intensive physiotherapy is required. Once again, the child may require inpatient supervision and recovery of knee function is slow. Scarring is often widened (Figure 7.9) and long-term patellar stability is not assured.

RECURRENT SUBLUXATION AND DISLOCATION

This disorder manifests towards the end of childhood and during adolescence. Girls are twice as commonly affected until the mid-teenage years when boys present more often. The dynamics of patellar tracking are usually demonstrably abnormal, although the changes may be subtle and best shown by computerized tomography (Fulkerson *et al.*, 1987). The classification of recurrent dislocation has been discussed by Jackson (1992) who divided the condition in the second and third decades of life into:

(i) lateral subluxation of the patella in extension

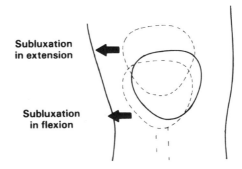

Figure 7.8 Subluxation may occur in extension, in flexion or in both positions, particularly if the patient is asked to exercise under load

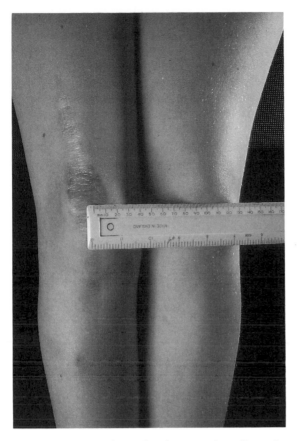

Figure 7.9 Widened scarring after quadriceps lengthening and patellar realignment. The right patella is at the end of the ruler while the left patella still lies proximal to the upper edge of the ruler

(ii) lateral subluxation in flexion
(iii) dislocation with no evidence of maltracking

A family history of patellofemoral problems is often present and internal torsion of the femur, with or without external torsion of the tibia, predisposes to instability by producing a large Q angle (Figure 7.10). The femoral sulcus may be shallow and a variety of patterns of patellofemoral incongruency have been described (Merchant *et al.*, 1974; Laurin *et al.*, 1979; Merchant, 1992). Genu valgum is no more common than in asymptomatic children.

The diagnosis is often missed by the inexperienced since episodes of giving way and medial discomfort are wrongly ascribed to meniscal pathology. The patella rarely presents in its dislocated position and an effusion is only seen acutely. The apprehension sign is positive, patellar manipulation is painful and the opposite knee may also be symptomatic. The patella may be laterally displaced or tilted on the skyline radiographic projection but variations in patellar shape do not appear to be of much consequence. The patellofemoral relationship in the first 30° of flexion is of significance, and avulsion and osteochondral fragments may be present.

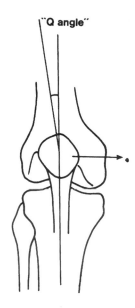

"Q angle"

Figure 7.10 The Q angle is formed by a line drawn from the anterior superior iliac spine to the centre of the patella, and a second line from that point to the tibial tuberosity. An increased angle may predispose the patella to lateral subluxation and therefore a medial vector of force, shown by the arrow, has to be provided by the vastus medialis muscle and patellar retinacular fibres

Direct trauma can, however, produce a dislocation in a normal knee, and this may be accompanied by a shearing, osteochondral fracture of the patella or the contiguous femoral condyle (Figure 7.11a,b). The patella usually dislocates laterally but may also jam inferiorly, superiorly or medially.

Indirect violence, for example when the patient twists on the weight-bearing leg, may be sufficient to cause an inherently weak patellofemoral articulation to dislocate spontaneously. Nevertheless, it is often difficult to state with certainty whether conditions such as patella alta, a shallow femoral groove, torsional abnormalities of the legs, ligament laxity or quadriceps weakness are directly responsible for the resultant instability of the patellofemoral joint.

After an acute lateral patellar dislocation a haemarthrosis develops, unless an extensive synovial tear has occurred, in which case the blood escapes to form a boggy and ill-defined haematoma. An arthroscopy should be combined with skyline views of the patella (see Chapter 3) in order to define the presence of an intra-articular fracture which may interfere with the later function of the patellofemoral joint. The medial retinacular fibres of the patella are invariably partially or completely ruptured, and the stretched vastus medialis muscle will be incompetent for several weeks.

TREATMENT OF ADOLESCENT PATELLAR INSTABILITY

Acute

Acute, traumatic dislocation is treated by a splint or brace initially, and aspiration of the haemarthrosis will lessen pain. Radiographs should be scrutinized for the presence of osteochondral injury, although the films are often of poor quality since the child is distressed.

Splintage for 4 weeks allows the torn medial retinaculum to heal with the minimum of lengthening. Surgical repair is unnecessary but the interior of the knee is examined arthroscopically if an osteochondral fragment is present. Since the medial capsule is breached, arthroscopic review should be delayed for 2 weeks. Some articular cartilage lesions may merit replacement and fixation, but usually the fragments are small and can be removed. Fibrin glue is unlikely to offer sufficient bonding of osteochondral fragments and therefore temporary fixation of larger fragments with K wires is appropriate. Rehabilitation is usually slow, with gradual resumption of the knee flexion and physiotherapy as described in Chapter 10. Vastus medialis tone (Figure 7.12) should stabilize patellar tracking in the majority of cases.

Chronic

If conservative measures fail to control patellar instability the patient will continue to experience regular episodes of locking and giving way, and less frequent complete patellar dislocation. A variety of proximal and distal realignment procedures have been described but it is important to define the nature of the patellar dislocation before deciding upon surgical correction. If the instability and lateral shift occur when the knee is extended lateral release will only worsen the tracking if it is not combined with distal

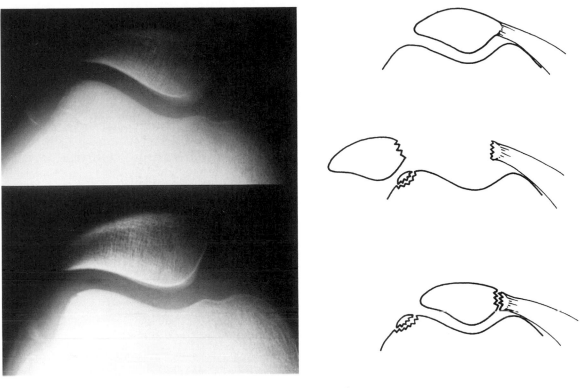

(a)   (b)

Figure 7.11 A lateral femoral condylar shear fracture (a) with a loose body that became fixed and enlarged with time (below). Medial avulsion (marginal) fracture of the patella may coexist (b)

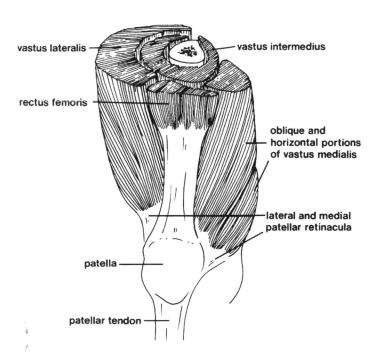

Figure 7.12 The control of patellar tracking depends upon the quadriceps muscle groups and the retinacular fibres

realignment of the patella. Recurrence of patellar instability is fairly common after surgery and recently Arnbjörnsson *et al.* (1992) reported the results of unilateral operation for bilateral patellar dislocation. At an average of 14 years after surgery they found that the surgically treated knee generally functioned worse than the conservatively managed joint, even though the preoperative problem was approximately the same on both sides. The rate of redislocation was reduced to around 5–10%, but at the expense of the later onset of osteoarthritis. Concerns about the induction of arthritic change were also expressed by Hampson and Hill (1975) and Barbari *et al.* (1990), where the danger of distal transfer of the tibial tuberosity was described, and by Crosby and Insall (1976) who advised against more than soft-tissue realignment. The frequency of patellar dislocation lessens with age (Larsen and Lauridsen, 1982) but is itself associated with the onset of mild patellofemoral degenerative change.

When repeated and disabling episodes of patellar dislocation are accompanied by effusions, and the child is severely restricted by the disability, a conservative policy of management should on rare occasions be abandoned. A simple lateral release for patellar dislocation in flexion may prove sufficient although this procedure alone affects patellar tracking very little since the reciprocal shapes of the patellar and femoral articular surfaces dictate in large measure the position of the patella during various stages of knee flexion.

Both proximal and distal surgical realignment of the patellar mechanism have been advocated, and sometimes a combination of these procedures is necessary (Figure 7.13). However, the variation in patellar morphology and uncertainty about the source of the symptoms that are produced by the patellofemoral joint make the outcome of surgery very unpredictable. In the absence of clearly identified patellar subluxation, surgery to the quadriceps muscle or patellar tendon should be avoided, as changes in the distribution and degree of loading on the knee cap will not necessarily prove beneficial.

A variety of proximal and distal realignment procedures have been described in association with a lateral release. Proximally, the vastus medialis can be plicated, and thus tightened; however, paradoxically, this may impair the function of that muscle and the surgeon must be at pains to avoid weakening the medial vector of force which controls patellar tracking. Various connective tissue structures, including the tendon of the semitendinosus muscle, can be used to medialize the position of the quadriceps mechanism. In time, any transferred connective tissue will tend to elongate and there may be no substantial improvement in patellar tracking. Once again, it should be recalled that muscle tone may be reduced by these procedures.

Distal realignment is a somewhat simpler technique, but the danger here lies in producing an excessive degree of medial and distal positioning of the patellar tendon. The Goldthwaite–Roux procedure employs only the lateral half of the patellar tendon, which is transposed beneath the medial half of the tendon and inserted into the inner side of the tibial tuberosity. A small block of bone can be removed to ensure good healing, although the use of a compression screw and washer is usually adequate. However, the presence of a screw at this rather sensitive site over the upper shin is often a source

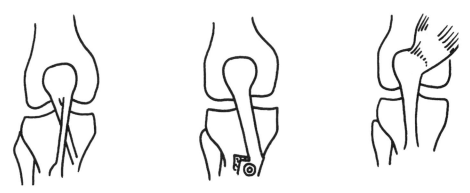

Figure 7.13 Distal patellar realignment is achieved by moving a lamina of the patellar tendon medially or by transposing the whole of the tuberosity medially after the end of skeletal growth. Proximal realignment employs some form of reefing, using vastus medialis or some other dynamic structure. An extensive lateral patellar release should accompany these procedures

of symptoms. Furthermore, scarring over the tibial tuberosity is usually tender for a prolonged period.

Procedures which move the whole insertion of the patellar tendon, including a block of bone, are now usually avoided. An excessive degree of distal as well as medial realignment produces osteoarthritis of the knee, and damage to the growth plate in the younger patient may result in a hyper-extension deformity of the proximal tibia (see Figure 4.5). The bone block procedure is therefore contraindicated in the adolescent. Both the proximal and distal soft-tissue procedures may be necessary where gross patellar instability is present, but there is always the risk that function may lessen and pain actually increase.

RETROPATELLAR PAIN SYNDROME

There is no one term that adequately and specifically defines this trouble-some condition which affects so many young people. The term 'chondro-malacia patellae' is inaccurate as it suggests that the articular surfaces of the patella and the associated femoral condyles are in some way softened or abnormal (Outerbridge, 1961; Abernethy *et al.*, 1978). This is very rarely the case in younger patients, and an absence of any characteristic cartilagi-nous lesion (Mori *et al.*, 1991) (Figure 7.14) has only highlighted the general dissatisfaction experienced by patient and doctor alike when dealing with this perplexing condition. The term 'anterior knee pain' is so bland and non-specific that it is perhaps preferable. The common sites where pain and tenderness are described (Figure 7.15) do not necessarily relate to structures directly at those localities and discomfort may be experienced at several places.

Patellar pain is produced by a large number of abnormalities (Fulkerson and Shea, 1990), some of which are related to the patella and others of which are distant to it (Table 7.1). It is therefore helpful to distinguish between pain and tenderness:

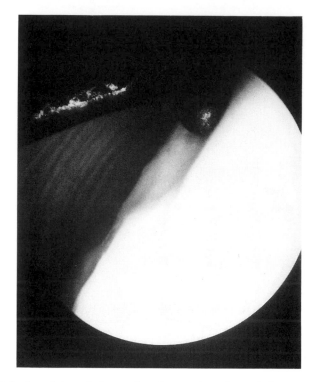

Figure 7.14 *Softening of the articular cartilage is a poorly understood phenomenon*

- Directly localized to the patella.
- Principally in parapatellar structures.
- Of a more generalized nature, but principally in the front of the knee

It must be remembered that the knee may be the site of referred pain from both the hip and back, and juvenile conditions affecting the hip commonly produce pain over the anterior and medial aspects of the knee.

Patellar pain is frequently seen in the child actively involved with sport. There is no convincing evidence that the symptoms worsen during a 'growth spurt', although there is no doubt that stress through the patellofemoral joint will increase from both overuse and rapid elongation of the lower limb. Milgrom *et al.* (1991) studied male army recruits prospectively and found that 15% developed anterior knee pain. The only predictive factors were isometric quadriceps strength, which rather confounds the basis of physiotherapy for this condition, and mild varus alignment.

Royle *et al.* (1991), in a prospective study of knee arthroscopy cases, found that 40% of patients without patellar pain presented with chondral fibrillation (Figure 7.16), whereas 40% with anterior symptoms had no patellar cartilage changes. The lack of correlation between the clinical symptoms and definable pathology has been appreciated for some time (Abernethy *et al.*, 1978) and therefore a large number of aetiological factors has been implicated (Table 7.1). Obvious osteochondral lesions are uncommon and the management of osteochondritis dissecans patellae (Figure 7.17) (Edwards and Bentley, 1977) follows the same principles of management as osteochondritis dissecans at other sites in the knee (Chapter 9).

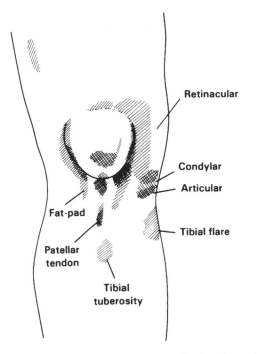

Figure 7.15 *The common sites of patellar pain are not confined to the patella and its synovial borders*

The problems associated with malalignment syndromes and variations in patellar shape, tracking and loading usually prove complex to understand, let alone to modify by operation, and the presence of ligament laxity adversely affects the surgical intentions of realignment (Insall, 1982).

Arnoldi (1991) has implicated an elevation of intraosseous venous pressure in patellar pain syndromes, similar to the disturbance in venous drainage seen in osteoarthritis. However, intraosseous phlebography is open to considerable errors in measurement and the significance of the alteration in patellar vascularity remains uncertain but intriguing. Similarly, the patterns of chondropathy (Mori *et al.*, 1991) do not correlate convincingly with observed symptoms.

Abnormalities in ossification, particularly of the superolateral secondary ossification centre of the patella, may also result in tenderness and pain in the region of the patella (Figure 7.18). At the end of skeletal growth the bipartite patella may become asymptomatic or may continue to cause disability (Weaver, 1977). Excision of one or more ununited fragments or lateral patellar release (Osborne and Fulford, 1982) will usually alleviate the pain. Acute, marginal fracture is easily distinguishable from bipartite patella but may confuse the unwary. Osteolytic lesions may occur as a result of neoplastic change (Linscheid and Dahlin, 1966), including chondroblastoma, giant cell tumour, aneurysmal bone cysts, plasmacytoma (McLeod and Macnicol, 1990) and metastases, and infection (Figure 7.19).

Other local abnormalities which should be considered include the presence of a plica, generally over the medial femoral condyle. The plica represents a hypertrophied synovial fold, and may be post-traumatic.

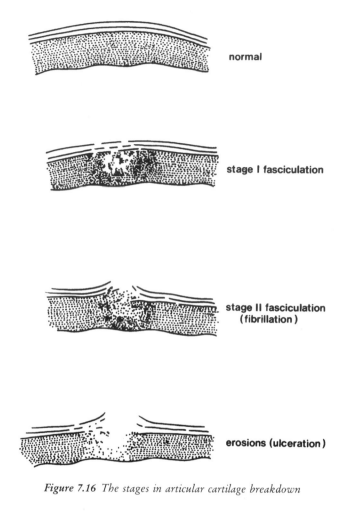

Figure 7.16 The stages in articular cartilage breakdown

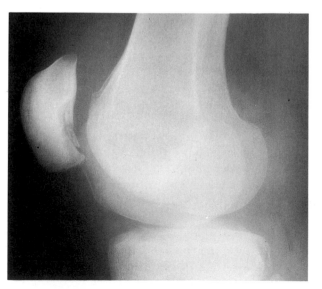

Figure 7.17 Osteochondritis dissecans patellae

Table 7.1 Different pathological conditions producing anterior knee pain

Site	Pathology
Patellar	Trauma (osteochondral fracture)
	Abnormal pressure or stress:
	(a) Increased or decreased
	(b) With or without patellofemoral instability
	(c) With or without patellar tilting
	Abnormal ossification centre
	Sinding–Larsen–Johansson syndrome
	Patellofemoral arthropathy
	'True' chondromalacia patellae
	Osteoarthritis
Peripatellar	Synovial fringe lesion
	Medial fat-pad syndrome
	Synovitis
	Loose body
	Plica syndrome
Quadriceps mechanism	Chronic quadriceps weakness
	Quadriceps tendon partial rupture
	'Jumper's knee' (patellar ligament tendonitis or partial tear)
	Ligament laxity
Superficial	Prepatellar, infrapatellar or suprapatellar bursitis
	Neuroma (especially of the infrapatellar branch of the saphenous nerve)
	Scarring
	Skin conditions
Other	Referred pain (meniscal tear, ligament rupture, hip pathology, lumbar disc herniation)
	Psychosomatic
	Idiopathic

Figure 2.8 shows the sites of the plicae which have been described, but these are generally only symptomatic when they enlarge to the extent that they rub against the femoral condyle or any other prominent bony margin of the knee. A contiguous lesion should therefore be identified over an articular surface, along with the thickened band (Figure 7.20). Fat-pad lesions (Hoffa, 1904) are rare and inferior pole tenderness is usually secondary to bursitis, patellar tendon avulsion (Sinding-Larsen, 1921) and other stress lesions of the patellar attachment (Figure 7.21).

A non-specific discomfort in the patellofemoral joint will occur after a patient has walked on a flexed knee, whatever the reason, for more than a few days. In the years of skeletal maturation, pain in and around the knee is quite common and may be due to 'growing pains'. These can be exacerbated by sport, where the patellofemoral mechanism, for example, is further stressed by strenuous activities. Generally, at the end of growth, any increase in the musculotendinous tension secondary to bone elongation will lessen and the pain should settle after one or two years.

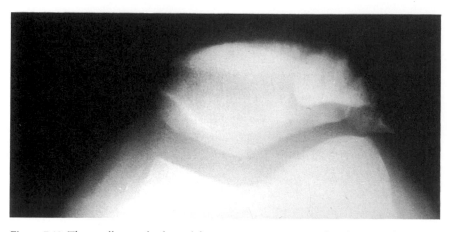

Figure 7.18 The patella may be formed from two or more centres of ossification which fail to coalesce

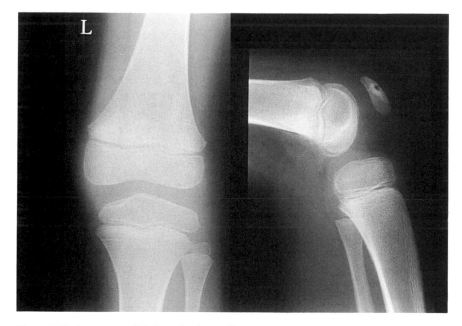

Figure 7.19 An osteomyelitic focus in the patella

However, other abnormalities must be ruled out, and this requires a careful history and investigation of the knee, including radiographs. It must never be forgotten that the cause of pain over the medial aspect of the knee may reside in the hip and, in any examination of the knee, the hip, spine and lower leg and foot should be carefully assessed. Referred pain in this manner, which radiates down a branch of the obturator nerve from the hip joint, occurs in cases of slipped epiphysis, Perthes' disease and osteonecrosis, septic and degenerative arthritis and in any other condition where the hip joint capsule is distended by an effusion. Thus, another common cause

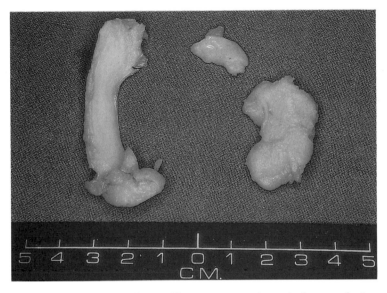

Figure 7.20 An excised plica which resembles a meniscus owing to its hypertrophy in response to chronic friction against the medial femoral condyle

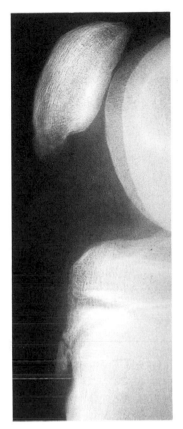

Figure 7.21 Sinding-Larsen–Johansson syndrome affecting the inferior patellar pole and a fracture of the tibial tuberosity

of knee pain occurs in the child with a transient synovitis of the hip, where symptoms may be felt over the medial aspect of the knee rather than proximally.

In many cases, retropatellar pain is apparently idiopathic. It is important to try to establish the cause if possible, and in this respect the age and sex of the patient, and also any abnormality of body build, should be noted. When examining the knee, particular attention should be given to patellar tracking, and the position of the patella both when the knee is fully extended and during flexion. The patient may walk with knee caps which squint inwards owing to persistent femoral anteversion, and there may be obvious knock-knee or other angulatory or torsional abnormalities. If the patient sits with the legs dangling over the edge of the examination couch, patellar tracking is readily observed under load as each knee in turn is straightened against gravity.

Investigations should include an arthroscopy in cases where the pain gives cause for concern, and the radiographs can be augmented by isotope bone scanning and CT scanning if this is felt to be necessary. However, in most cases of patellar pain a careful physical examination is all that is required (Ficat and Hungerford, 1977; Bentley and Dowd, 1984). Arthroscopy will fail to detect changes deep to the articular cartilage (Imai and Tomatsu, 1991) and the expense of MR scanning is such that it should only be used in the chronic and unresponsive case.

Treatment of patellar pain

Symptoms in adolescence tend to remit with time, although Karlstrom (1940) found that after 20 years many patients were still symptomatic. Sandow and Goodfellow (1985) reported that counselling and physiotherapy alleviated the symptoms in half of a group of adolescent girls, although symptoms persisted in the rest. In a prospective study of 30 adolescents, O'Neill *et al.* (1992) found that symptomatic relief was achieved in 85% of cases by isometric quadriceps and hamstring strengthening coupled with iliotibial band stretching. McConnell (1986) has also popularized the conservative approach to anterior knee pain (see Chapter 10) and presumably these alterations in loading at the patellofemoral joint reduce shear and compressive forces to which the patella is subjected. The effects of physiotherapy may be short-lived, particularly if the exercise programme is abandoned. Yet the conservative approach at least succeeds in demonstrating that the symptoms can be controlled by conscious effort in the majority of patients.

Lateral patellar release is recommended less frequently for patellar pain than used to be the case (Osborne and Fulford, 1982). The indiscriminate use of this release was based on the mistaken belief that the procedure was a safe and benign intervention, particularly if carried out arthroscopically. Hughston and Deese (1989) described the risk of producing medial patellar subluxation postoperatively if the vastus lateralis is wasted, and haemarthrosis, reflex sympathetic dystrophy and painful clicking at the lateral patellar edge may complicate the operation. Demonstrable tightness of the lateral parapatellar tissues and an absence of patellar hypermobility were considered to be important preconditions of successful lateral patellar release by Gecha and Torg (1990), and Fulkerson and Shea (1990) have stressed the importance of identifying the lateral retinaculum as pathologically tight before interfering with a structure which balances the patella during tracking.

Lateral release also offers an analgesic effect but the results are unpredictable, so that after two or three years there is a return of symptoms in a substantial portion of patients. Denervation of the lateral capsule has been shown to occur anatomically (Abraham *et al.*, 1989) and reinnervation may account for the resumption of symptoms.

When severe patellar pain persists after lateral patellar release, and in the absence of any intra-articular knee pathology or alternative disease process, the Maquet procedure and patellar osteotomy (Morscher, 1980; Macnicol, 1985, 1994) have been proposed as alternatives to patellectomy. If there seems to be an 'excess' of retropatellar pressure, such as when sitting or climbing stairs, then there may be a place for raising the patella anteriorly away from the femoral groove. Maquet has suggested an operation where the distal tibial attachment is elevated, in the belief that a 1 cm shift of the tuberosity anteriorly reduces patellar pressure by 20–40%. However, this concept is based upon cadaveric studies, and the dynamics of the patellofemoral joint following this procedure in the living are unknown. There is also the risk that moving the patella anteriorly will increase its likelihood of either subluxing or tilting laterally, and the prominence of the tibial tuberosity postoperatively may adversely affect wound healing and leave the proximal shin significantly tender.

An alternative approach has been to recommend a patellectomy for cases of intractable anterior knee pain. This does not guarantee success, and extension of the knee is weakened by at least 15%. Paradoxically the anterior knee pain regularly persists in the absence of the patella. In order

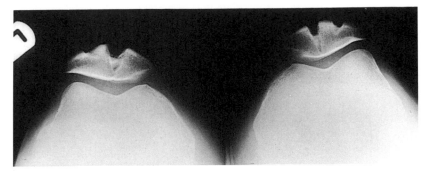

Figure 7.22 Patellar sagittal osteotomy for intractable anterior knee pain

to preserve the patella, a patellar osteotomy may be of value in these very difficult cases and it is of interest to note that the cancellous bone of the patella often appears very dry and avascular during this procedure, suggesting that an 'osteodystrophy' is responsible for the anterior knee pain in a proportion of cases. However, the osteotomy may hasten osteoarthritic changes in the patellofemoral joint, if it breaches the subchondral plate, and only a sagittal cut should be utilized so that proximal patellar blood supply is not impaired (Scapinelli, 1967) (Figure 7.22).

Whichever surgical procedure is recommended, the surgeon must be aware of the complications that may ensue and the fact that many patients will respond poorly to an operation which addresses a syndrome where the cause of the symptoms is still so little understood. If surgery is advised it should only be after a prolonged period of physiotherapy, possibly with some form of supportive bracing for the knee cap, and a modification of activities.

It is also important to stress to the patient, and the parents, that anterior knee pain, from whatever cause, may have to be accepted, and that there may be a slight but never complete lessening in symptoms with time. The use of anti-inflammatory analgesics over a prolonged period is inadvisable, although there was a vogue for salicylate therapy used for short periods. If the anxiety of the patient (and parent) can be reduced, and an acceptable level of sporting activity prescribed, many patients seem quite ready to live within the limits set by their patellofemoral symptoms. As a general rule, surgery should be conservative and restricted to soft tissue only in the growing child.

Thereafter, any procedure which is directed towards the articular cartilage must be justified carefully, and it is probably better to confine surgery to a distal realignment procedure where patellar maltracking is obvious or to, at most, a patellar osteotomy in those with no obvious abnormality of patellar movement. Patellectomy should be avoided if at all possible, particularly as osteoarthritis of the knee will be hastened, yet there is a small group of patients who seem to benefit from patellectomy and the difficulty lies in defining this group. Resurfacing operations for the patellofemoral joint are still experimental and they have no place as yet in the management of the younger patient.

Sinding-Larsen–Johansson's disease

Pain over the lower pole of the patella may be associated with a small avulsion of bone (Sinding-Larsen, 1921). In rare cases an ossicle forms and the symptoms persist. The combination of rapid growth and repetitive sport triggers this overuse syndrome which is seen most commonly between the ages of 9 and 14 years. Rest is all that is required in the majority of cases, and it is preferable to avoid the use of a plaster cylinder. Local ultrasound and the application of a non-steroidal anti-inflammatory gel may lessen the discomfort and the child and parents should be reassured that the condition will heal slowly. In rare instances the attachment to the inferior patellar pole merits drilling and a mobile ossicle should be excised if it is painful when manipulated. The acute sleeve fracture (Houghton and Ackroyd, 1979) should be suspected when sudden pain ocurs at the lower pole; radiographs are diagnostic, although X-rays rarely show the true size of the separated osteochondral fragment.

Osgood–Schlatter's disease

This common complaint was described separately by Osgood and Schlatter in 1903. Ogden and Southwick (1976) reviewed the developmental changes in the tuberosity with growth, and the pattern of ossification. Under the stress of skeletal growth and active sport the preosseous cartilage is partially avulsed and the trauma leads to hypertrophy (see Plate 30). Boys are affected three times more commonly than girls and the contralateral tuberosity may become symptomatic 6–18 months later in approximately a quarter of cases. Once again it is most common in late childhood and usually resolves during adolescence, leaving variable enlargement of the tendon insertion. It affects athletic youngsters (Kujala *et al.*, 1985) and hypertrophy of both it and Gerdy's tubercle are seen in many sprinters, soccer players and gymnasts.

A reduction in sport and counselling about the temporary nature of the condition is usually all that is required, although symptoms persist for several years in most patients. Kneeling and squatting are avoided by the patient quite naturally, and local treatment may be helpful but only gives short-term relief. Splintage should be used sparingly as there is a risk that the introspective child will develop more morbid symptoms.

If an ossicle develops in adolescence (see Figure 4.2) its excision may relieve the symptoms although this is by no means assured. Drilling of the tuberosity, and partial reduction of its size, are more speculative procedures, occasionally advocated if disabling symptoms persist. As with any anterior knee pain syndrome, surgical intervention should never be considered before a period of conservative treatment.

Patellar tendonitis

Tenderness in relation to the patellar tendon is usually localized to one or other end of the tendon in childhood. This differs from the adults where symptoms occur from a prepatellar or infrapatellar bursitis, or from a similar inflammatory process between the tendon and the upper tibia. Blazina *et al.*

(1973) coined the phrase 'jumper's knee' for a variety of conditions that affect the patellar tendon and its attachments. Overuse, particularly repetitive eccentric loading, triggers symptoms which may be present bilaterally in approximately 20% of patients. Inflammatory changes results from microtrauma either in the tendon or at its interface with bone. Cystic changes may become apparent using ultrasound examination (Fritschy and De Gautard, 1988) and the tendon later feels thickened as fibrosis develops. The pathological changes can also be detected by MR scanning.

Rest and anti-inflammatory agents are usually prescribed, but enforced inactivity is rarely acceptable to the elite athlete. Changes in training technique and orthotic adjustment of the shoes may help those involved with basketball, volleyball and athletics, but the symptoms persist in a proportion. Sometimes a leg-length discrepancy is evident and should be corrected by a contralateral shoe insert. Steroid injection is not advisable because of the risks of worsening the lesion, so that surgical exploration is the only effective recourse in the chronic case (Colosimo and Bassett, 1990). This helps to relieve any constriction and rekindles the healing process. Excision and detachment of portions of the tendon is illogical and risky, but excision of a bursitis is effective.

References

Abernethy, P.J., Townsend, P.R., Rose, R.M. and Radin, E.L. (1978) Is chondromalacia patellae a separate clinical entity? *J. Bone Joint Surg.*, **60B**, 205–210

Abraham, E., Washington, E. and Huang, T.-L. (1989) Insall proximal realignment for disorders of the patella. *Clin. Orthop.*, **248**, 61–65

Arnbjörnsson, A., Egund, N., Rydling, O. *et al.* (1992) The natural history of recurrent dislocation of the patella. *J. Bone Joint Surg.*, **74B**, 140–142

Arnoldi, C.C. (1991) The patellar pain syndrome. *Acta Orthop. Scand.*, **62**(Suppl.), 1–29

Barbari, S., Raugstad, T.S., Lichtenberg, N. and Refrem, D. (1990) The Hauser operation for patellar dislocation. *Acta Orthop. Scand.*, **61**, 32–35

Bentley, G. and Dowd, G. (1984) Current concepts in the etiology and treatment of chondromalacia patellae. *Clin. Orthop.*, **189**, 209–228

Blackburne, J.S. and Peel, T.E. (1977) A new method of measuring patellar height. *J. Bone Joint Surg.*, **59B**, 241–242

Blazina, M.E., Kerlan, R.K., Jobe, F.W. *et al.* (1973) Jumper's knee. *Orthop. Clin. N. Am.*, **4**, 665–678

Blumensaat, C. (1932) Die Lageabweichungen und verrenkungen der kniescheibe. *Ergebn. Chir. Orthop.*, **31**, 149–223

Carter, C.O. (1960) Recurrent dislocation of the patella and of the shoulder. *J. Bone Joint Surg.*, **42B**, 721–727

Colosimo, A.J. and Bassett, F.H. (1990) Jumper's knee : diagnosis and treatment. *Orthop. Rev.*, **19**, 139–149

Crosby, E.B. and Insall, J. (1976) Recurrent dislocation of the patella : relation of treatment to osteoarthritis. *J. Bone Joint Surg.*, **58A**, 9–13

Edwards, D.H. and Bentley, G. (1977) Osteochondritis dissecans patellae. *J. Bone Joint Surg.*, **59B**, 58–61

Ficat, R.P. and Hungerford, D.S. (1977) *Disorders of the Patellofemoral Joint*, Williams and Wilkins, Baltimore

Fritschy, D. and De Gautard, R. (1988) Jumper's knee and ultrasonography. *Am. J. Sports Med.*, **16**, 637–640

Fulkerson, J.P., Schutzer, S.F., Ramsby, G.R. and Bernstein, R.A. (1987) Computerised tomography of the patellofemoral joint before and after lateral release or realignment. *Arthroscopy*, **3**, 19–24

Fulkerson, J.P. and Shea, K.P. (1990) Current concepts review : disorders of patellofemoral alignment. *J. Bone Joint Surg.*, **72A**, 1424–1429

Gecha, S.R. and Torg, J.S. (1990) Clinical prognosticators for the efficacy of retinacular release surgery to treat patellofemoral pain. *Clin. Orthop.*, **253**, 203–208

Goa, G.-X., Lee, E.H. and Bose, K. (1990) Surgical management of congenital and habitual dislocation of the patellae. *J. Pediatr. Orthop.*, **10**, 255–260

Gunn, D.R. (1964) Contracture of the quadriceps muscle. *J. Bone Joint Surg.*, **46B**, 492–497

Hampson, W.G.J. and Hill, P. (1975) Late results of transfer of the tibial tubercle for recurrent dislocation of the patella. *J. Bone Joint Surg.*, **57B**, 209–213

Hoffa, A. (1904) The influence of the adipose tissue with regard to the pathology of the knee joint. *J. Am. Med. Ass.*, **43**, 795–796

Houghton, G.R. and Ackroyd, C.E. (1979) Sleeve fractures of the patellar in children. *J. Bone Joint Surg.*, **61B**, 165

Hughston, J.C. and Deese, M. (1989) Medial subluxation of the patella as a complication of lateral retinacular release. *Adv. Orthop. Surg.*, **12**, 170–171

Imai, N. and Tomatsu, T. (1991) Cartilage lesions in the knee of adolescents and young adults : arthroscopic analysis. *Arthroscopy*, **7**, 198–203

Insall, J. (1982) Current concepts review : patellar pain. *J. Bone Joint Surg.*, **64A**, 147–152

Insall, J. and Salvati, E. (1971) Patella position in the normal knee joint. *Radiology.*, **101**, 101–104

Jackson, A.M. (1992) Recurrent dislocation of the patella. *J. Bone Joint Surg.*, **74B**, 2–4

Karlstrom, S. (1940) Chondromalacia patellae. *Acta Chir. Scand.*, **64**, 347–381

Kujala, V., Kuist, M. and Heinonen, O. (1985) Osgood–Schlatter's disease in adolescent athletes. *Am. J. Sports Med.*, **13**, 236–241

Larsen, E. and Lauridsen, F. (1982) Conservative treatment of patella dislocations. *Clin. Orthop.*, **171**, 131–136

Laurin, C.A., Dussault, R. and Levesque, H.P. (1979) The tangential x-ray investigation of the patellofemoral joint. *Clin. Orthop.*, **144**, 16–26

Linscheid, R.L. and Dahlin, D.C. (1966) Unusual lesions of the patella. *J. Bone Joint Surg.*, **48A**, 1359–1366

McConnell, J. (1986) The management of chondromalacia patellae : a long-term solution. *Aust. J. Physiother.*, **32**, 215–220

McLeod, G.C. and Macnicol, M.F. (1990) Plasmacytoma of the patella. *J. Roy. Coll. Surg. Edinb.*, **35**, 195–196

Macnicol, M.F. (1985) Patellar osteotomy for intractable anterior knee pain. *J. Bone Joint Surg.*, **67B**, 156

Macnicol, M.F. (1994) Patellar osteotomy for intractable patellar pain. *The Knee*, **1**, 41–45

Merchant, A.C. (1992) Radiologic evaluation of the patellofemoral joint. In *Knee Surgery* (eds Aichroth, P.M. and Cannon, W.D.), Martin Dunitz, London, pp. 380–388

Merchant, A.C., Mercer, R.L., Jacobsen, R.H. and Cool, C.R. (1974) Roentgenographic analysis of paellofemoral congruence. *J. Bone Joint Surg.*, **56A**, 1391–1396

Milgrom, C., Finestone, A., Eldad, A. and Shlamkovitch, N. (1991) Patellofemoral pain caused by overactivity : a prospective study of risk factors in infantry recruits. *J. Bone Joint Surg.*, **73A**, 1041–1043

Mori, Y., Kuroki, Y., Yamamoto, R. *et al.* (1991) Clinical and histological study of patellar chondropathy in adolescents. *Arthroscopy*, **7**, 182–197

Morscher, E. and Dick, W. (1980) Sagittal patellar osteotomy in chondromalacia patellae. *Orthop. Prax.*, **16**, 692–695

Ogden, J.A. and Southwick, W.O. (1976) Osgood–Schlatter's disease and tibial tuberosity development. *Clin. Orthop.*, **116**, 180–186

O'Neill, D.B., Micheli, L.J. and Warner, J.P. (1992) Patellofemoral stress : a prospective analysis of exercise treatment in adolescents and adults. *Am. J. Sports Med.*, **20**, 151–156

Osborne, A.H. and Fulford, P.C. (1982) Lateral release for chondromalacia patellae. *J. Bone Joint Surg.*, **64B**, 202–205

Outerbridge, R.E. (1961) The aetiology of chondromalacia patellae. *J. Bone Joint Surg.*, **43B**, 313–321

Royle, S.G., Noble, J., Davies, D.R.A. and Kay, P.R. (1991) The significance of chondromalacic changes on the patella. *Arthroscopy*, **7**, 158–160

Sandow, M.J. and Goodfellow, J.W. (1985) The natural history of anterior knee pain in adolescents. *J. Bone Joint Surg.*, **67B**, 36–39

Scapinelli, R. (1967) Blood supply of the human patella. *J. Bone Joint Surg.*, **44B**, 563–571

Sinding-Larsen, M.F. (1921) A hitherto unknown affection of the patella in children. *Acta Radiol.*, **1**, 171–175

Weaver, J.K. (1977) Bipartite patellae as the cause of disability in the athlete. *Am. J. Sports Med.*, **5**, 137–143

Williams, P.F. (1968) Quadriceps contracture. *J. Bone Joint Surg.*, **50B**, 278–284

Yates, C.K. and Grana, W.K. (1990) Patellofemoral pain in children. *Clin. Orthop.*, **255**, 36–43.

8
Fractures around the knee

INITIAL TREATMENT – PRINCIPLES OF FRACTURE CARE –
TIBIAL FRACTURES – FEMORAL FRACTURES – PATELLAR
FRACTURES – OSTEOCHONDRAL FRACTURES – EPIPHYSEAL
FRACTURES – STRESS FRACTURES – COMPLICATIONS OF
FRACTURES

Fractures involving the knee are relatively common, and often involve the articular surface of the joint. In childhood and old age the bone may yield before any major ligament tear occurs, whereas in the adult a ligament disruption commonly accompanies the fracture.

INITIAL TREATMENT

When a significant and unstable fracture has been sustained, the early management should include emergency splintage of the limb, appropriate surgical care of any wound, and attention to other injuries. If a fracture around the knee is associated with multiple injuries, then the patient will require resuscitation with blood transfusion and electrolyte solutions and the primary aim should be to ensure that there is no life-threatening condition. Unfortunately, serious injuries to the knee may be overlooked, or their treatment delayed, when a patient is admitted with multiple injuries. In addition, if displaced fractures of the femur or tibia have been sustained, the assessment of any ligamentous or bony damage around the knee may prove difficult.

PRINCIPLES OF FRACTURE CARE

The four Rs of fracture care are as follows:

- *Respect* the soft tissues, remembering that the blood supply to bone is reliant upon their integrity, as is wound healing
- *Reduce* the fracture, and maintain this reduction by external splintage, traction, internal fixation or possibly external fixation
- *Restore* function by ensuring that fixation of the fracture is adequate and that joint movement can be regained as rapidly as possible
- *Remember* that one is dealing with the whole patient. The emotional, social and economic concerns of the patient must be dealt with as effectively as possible, and every effort should be made to motivate the patient towards a successful recovery.

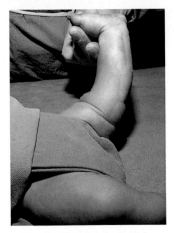

Plate 24 Congenital dislocation of the knee; the shortened quadriceps hold the knee hyperextended to a varying degree and flexion is restricted

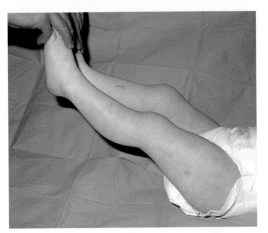

Plate 25 A locked right knee secondary to a torn discoid lateral meniscus

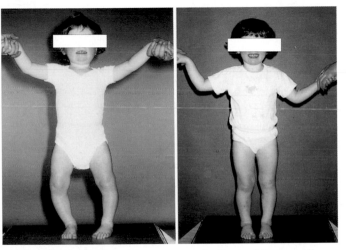

Plate 26 Constitutional genu varum in the toddler usually corrects before 5 years (right) Blount's disease is extremely rare (p 170)

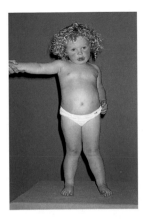

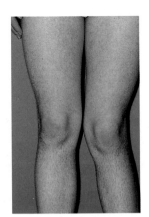

Plate 27(a) Constitutional genu valgum is particularly common in girls and is associated with generalized ligament laxity, femoral anteversion and protective intoeing. The condition becomes less obvious by later childhood

Plate 27(b) Post-traumatic genu valgum of the left knee (see also Fig 8.17)

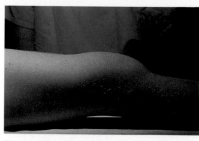

Plate 28 Generalized swelling of the knee in juvenile chronic arthritis

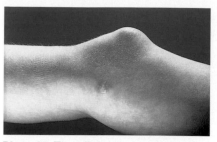

Plate 29 The discrete swelling of prepatellar bursitis ('housemaid's knee')

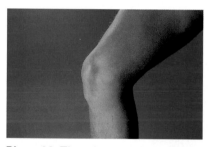

Plate 30 The popliteal cyst in childhood usually disappears

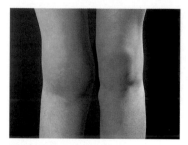

Plate 31 A left quadriceps ganglion

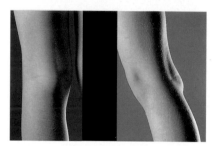

Plate 32 The characteristic bony lump of Osgood-Schlatter's disease

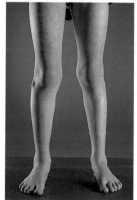

Plate 33 Chronic sub-luxation of the right fibular head. Surgery is rarely appropriate

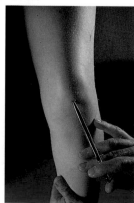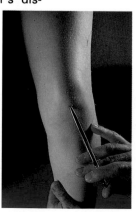

Plate 34 The left patella lies above the femoral sulcus but is centrally positioned

Plate 35 On contracting the quadriceps (or flexing the knee) the patella shifts laterally

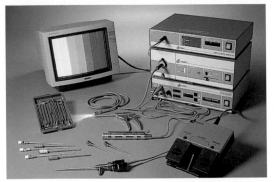

Plate 36 The Dyonics camera system and disposable shavers

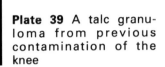

Plate 37 A smaller diameter arthroscope for paediatric use

Plate 38 The medial meniscus in a 4-year-old child's knee. Early pannus is present over the anterior and peripheral portion of the meniscus

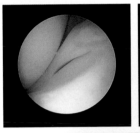

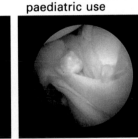

Plate 39 A talc granuloma from previous contamination of the knee

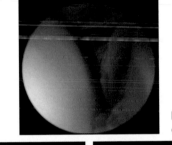

Plate 40 Arthroscopic appearance of synovitis

Plate 41 An osteochondral fracture of the medial femoral condyle

Plate 42 A loose body secondary to osteochondritis dissecans

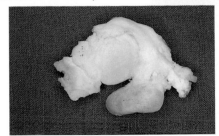

Plate 43 A discoid lateral meniscus with mucoid, cystic degeneration

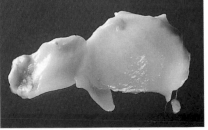

Plate 44 The Wrisberg type of discoid lateral meniscus (see p 108)

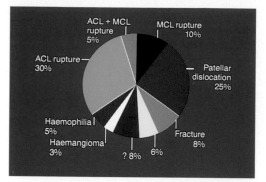

Plate 45 Causes of haemarthrosis of the knee in 55 children over a 10-year period. The yellow segment indicates synovial tears with no obvious associated pathology and the black segment four cases where no cause was found

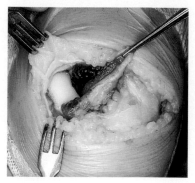

Plate 46 Haemangioma of the fat-pad producing repeated haemarthroses

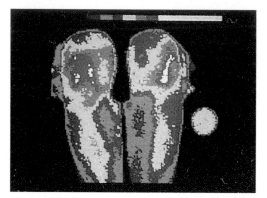

Plate 47 Chronic synovitis produces increased heat emission on thermography

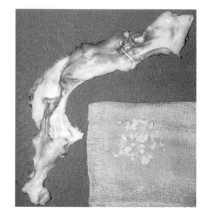

Plate 48 Synovial chondromatosis with a segment of hypertrophic synovium

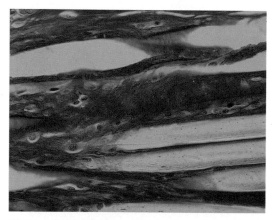

Plate 49 Collagen fibres forming along strands of the Leeds-Keio artificial ligament

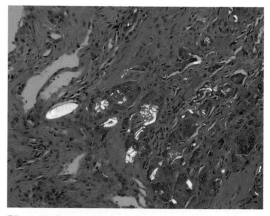

Plate 50 Foreign body inflammatory response surrounding fragments of artificial ligament

TIBIAL FRACTURES

Undisplaced fractures are best treated conservatively by plaster and then cast bracing (Hohl and Luck, 1956), although the displacement of fragments may be underestimated radiographically. Table 8.1 details the classic descriptive terminology for these tibial plateaux fractures. The AO group (Müller *et al.*, 1988) have produced their universal grouping as follows:

A   extra-articular
B_1 pure split
B_2 pure depression
B_3 split and depression
C_1 simple articular and simple metaphyseal
C_2 simple articular and multifragmentary metaphyseal
C_3 multifragmentary or comminuted

Roughly three-quarters of all fractures are in the B category (Figure 8.1a,b) and much debate centres on the acceptable level of displacement. Porter (1970) showed that fibrocartilage will fill in moderate splits and depressions, and early movement (Apley, 1956) has long been recommended to preserve range of motion and the joint surfaces. Fixation after reduction should be attempted with greater than 7 mm depression (Rasmussen and Sörensen, 1973) and depends upon the experience and skills of the surgeon (Burri *et al.*, 1979; Schatzker *et al.*, 1979). Arthroscopic review of the joint surfaces will help to monitor reduction of splitting or

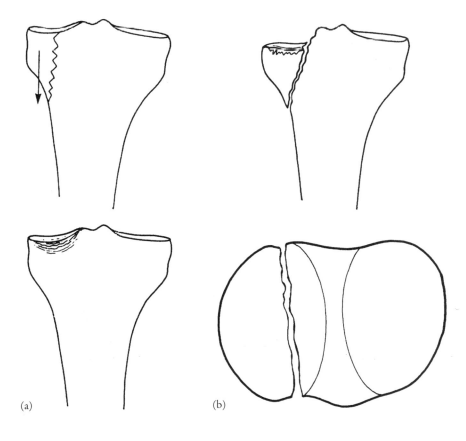

(a)   (b)

Figure 8.1 Minimally displaced type B tibial condylar fractures, (pure split above and partial depression below) (a) and displaced split and depression fractures (b)

depressed plateau fractures (O'Dwyer and Bobic, 1992) and meniscal inter-position. Meniscal tears are reported in varying degree (17–85%) and peripheral separations should certainly be repaired.

The C group of fractures involve the tibial condyles and were previously described by Schatzker *et al.* (1979) as medial condylar (type IV), lateral condylar with valgus tilting (type V) and bicondylar (type VI). Honkonen and Järvinen (1992) subdivided the bicondylar group into those tilted medially and those tilted laterally, believing that fixation and prognosis were different.

Ligament injuries are unusual, and difficult to treat in association with major joint surface displacement (Porter, 1970). Laxity is usually the result of split/depression fractures and proves very disabling. Osteoarthritis corre-lates with malalignment, pathological laxity and extensive articular involve-ment, especially if there has been significant loss of meniscal substance. Knee replacement may be appropriate in elderly patients with severe fracture patterns but the long-term outcome is not yet known.

Femoral shaft fractures are also accompanied by a significant incidence of knee injuries, Vangsness *et al.* (1993) finding at arthroscopy that complex and radial tears of the medial and lateral menisci were present in over 25% of patients. Almost half their cases demonstrated ligament laxity, although not necessarily in association with meniscal damage. A large portion of these lesions heal or become asymptomatic, but knee injury should always be assessed in patients with femoral fractures and with high-velocity tibial or hindfoot injuries.

FEMORAL FRACTURES

Fracture patterns of the distal femur are described in Table 8.1. The AO classification (Müller *et al.*, 1988) prefers the use of a coding system which can be applied universally as follows:

A_1 extra-articular – simple
A_2 extra-articular – metaphyseal wedge
A_3 extra-articular – metaphyseal complex
B_1 partially articular – lateral condylar sagittal
B_2 partially articular – medial condylar sagittal
B_3 partially articular – condylar in the frontal plane
C_1 completely articular - articular simple, metaphyseal simple
C_2 completely articular - articular simple, metaphyseal multifragmentary
C_3 multifragmentary

Although fractures of the femoral condyles can be treated with traction (Rockwood and Green, 1991) it is impossible to ensure precise reduction. Internal fixation is advised if facilities permit (Figure 8.2a,b), especially when displacement is major, when the fracture is irreducible, often due to soft-tissue interposition and the forces at play, and when a significant neurovascular deficit is present. Olerud (1972) presented one of the first major series of operative fixation, although the infection rate was up to 5%. Non-union can be avoided completely by anatomical reduction (Giles *et al.*, 1982) and Siliski *et al.* (1989) stressed the importance of avoiding resid-ual varus and internal deformities of the distal segment (Figure 8.3).

Table 8.1 Fractures involving the knee

Patellar		
Osteochondral	Medial avulsion	
	Lateral shear	
	Central shear	
Transverse	Undisplaced	
	Displaced	
Polar	Upper	
	Lower (including cartilaginous 'sleeve' fracture in child)	
Vertical		
Comminuted		
Tibial		
Plateau	Undisplaced:	
	a) Medial–anterior, posterior or total	
	b) Lateral–anterior, posterior or total	
	c) Comminuted medial and lateral	
	Displaced:	
	a) Split (single fragment)–sagittal or coronal; vertical or oblique	
	b) Compression (more than 3 mm depression of the articular surface)*	
	c) Split-compression	
	d) Comminuted	
Intercondylar eminence (including tibial spines)	Tilted up anteriorly:	
	a) Minor displacement	
	b) Major displacement	
	Complete separation:	
	a) No rotation	
	b) Rotated	
Tuberosity	Undisplaced	
	Displaced	
	Comminuted	
Femoral		
Supracondylar	Undisplaced:	*Anterior, posterior, marginal, central or total – use tomography with the film directed 15 degrees distally and centred over the knee joint since the slope of the plateaux to the tibial shaft is 105 degrees (otherwise the amount of depression is falsely magnified if there is a posterior depression, and underestimated for a central or anterior depression).
	a) Transverse	
	b) T or Y configuration	
	Impacted	
	Displaced:	
	a) Transverse	
	b) T or Y configuration	
	Comminuted	
Condylar	Undisplaced:	Open reduction if more than 20 degrees coronal tilting with the knee flexed approximately 20 degrees, or depression of the joint surface of 5 mm or more.
	a) Medial	
	b) Lateral	
	c) Both condyles	
	Displaced:	
	a) Medial	
	b) Lateral	
	c) Both condyles	
	Coronal	

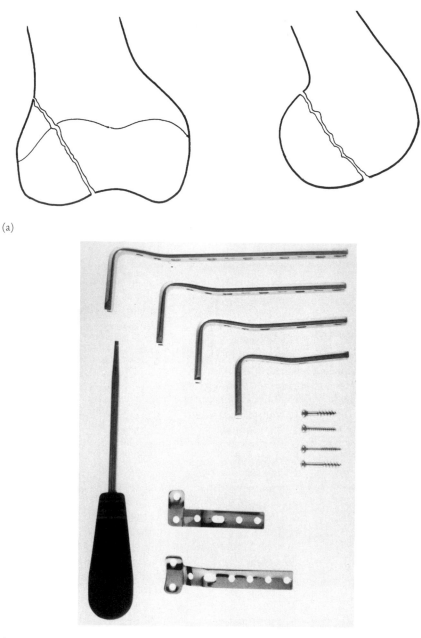

(a)

(b)

Figure 8.2 *Condylar fractures of the distal femur may occur in different planes (a). AO screws, blade plates and buttress plates offer an excellent means of fixation (b)*

A lateral incision and 95° AO blade plate (Müller *et al.*, 1970) or Richards device permit good fixation in the majority of cases, augmented with further intercondylar compression screws as necessary. Sanders *et al.* (1991) recommended the use of double plating, adding a medial buttress plate, for comminuted, unstable fractures. Stability should then allow early movement, although the soft-tissue dissection may result in stiffening from

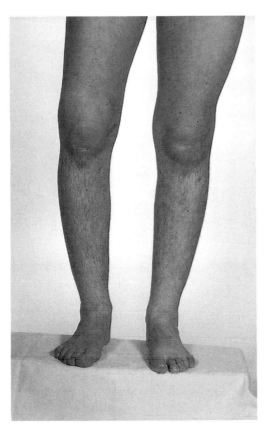

Figure 8.3 Residual varus after poor fixation of a left distal femoral fracture

adhesions. An interlocking intramedullary nail has a role in some supra-condylar and extensive intercondylar fractures (Leung *et al.*, 1992). Bone grafting and the impaction of metaphyseal bone in the elderly should ensure that non-union is minimal.

Active and passive movement of the knee is encouraged immediately postoperatively, and continuous passive motion is beneficial. Progressive weightbearing is encouraged and union is usually complete by the fourth month after injury.

With both tibial and femoral fractures, serious vascular or neurological injuries may coexist at the level of the knee. It is then advisable to fix the fracture internally at an early stage of management so that any vessel repair can be protected. After neurological injury, either to the leg itself or in the wider context of a patient with a major head injury, rehabilitation will be more rapid if the fracture is operated upon, although the risks of infection must always be balanced against the advantages of early and anatomical restoration of the fractured bone.

PATELLAR FRACTURES

Fractures of the patella are described in Table 8.1. Sometimes a secondary ossification centre is confused with an acute fracture, although the outline

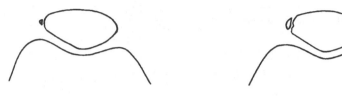

Avulsion of a portion of the medial retinacular attachment

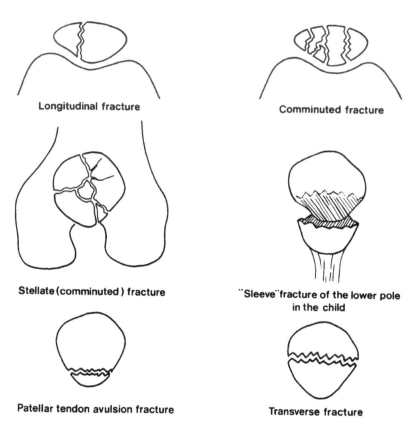

Longitudinal fracture

Comminuted fracture

Stellate (comminuted) fracture

"Sleeve" fracture of the lower pole in the child

Patellar tendon avulsion fracture

Transverse fracture

Figure 8.4 The different types of patellar fracture

of the former is always smooth and rounded and does not resemble the appearances after acute injury. Avulsion fractures of the patella (Dowd, 1982) may occur after a lateral patellar dislocation (Figure 8.4) and there may be associated shearing fractures of the osteochondral surfaces of the posterior patella (Figure 8.5).

A sudden contraction of the quadriceps muscle, in the absence of any direct injury to the front of the knee, may produce a transverse fracture of the patella which may be either undisplaced or displaced. In the child, such an avulsion fracture, involving the lower pole of the patella, pulls off a 'sleeve' of cartilage. This fragment may look innocuous radiographically,

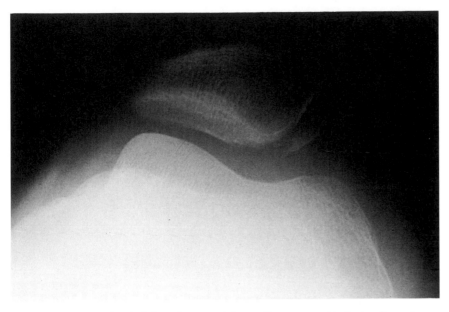

Figure 8.5 An osteochondral shear fracture of the patella seen on a 'skyline' radiograph

but constitutes a reason for internal fixation of what then turns out to be a fairly major fragment.

Where the patellar fracture is relatively simple, with either a major transverse or vertical component to it, internal fixation with circumferential wires and a tension band wiring system is recommended. This allows early movement of the knee and should restore the posterior articular surface of the patella. Injury to the articular surface of the femoral groove may coexist and will obviously have an adverse effect upon subsequent patellofemoral function.

The comminuted patellar fracture is best treated by early excision of the fragments. An attempt can be made to reduce the fragments and produce a reasonably articular surface, but this must be reviewed at the time of surgery and if incongruencies exist, then a patellectomy is more likely to relieve the patient of symptoms than a united but abnormal patella. Patellectomy results in some loss of knee extensor power, but if the medial and lateral retinacular fibres are carefully repaired and the capsule of the patella sutured to form a ligamentous structure, the end results of patellectomy are acceptable.

OSTEOCHONDRAL FRACTURES

Osteochondral and chondral fractures occur frequently in relation to the patellofemoral joint, as a result of lateral patellar dislocations. Very rarely, the tibial plateau may also be the site of such a fracture.

If these separation fragments are small, they can be removed arthroscopically (Hubbard, 1987). Larger fragments may be worth preserving, particularly if there is a bleeding base of cancellous bone (Figure 8.6). The use of 'fibrin glue' has been advocated as a means of fixing the small fragments in place, allied to a period of knee splintage. When fragments do

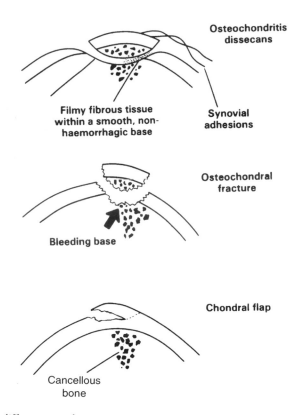

Figure 8.6 *The differentiation between osteochondritis dissecans, osteochondral fracture and a chondral flap*

not heal back adequately, they will separate and produce a loose body in the joint (Dandy, 1992).

Alternative forms of fixation of larger osteochondral fractures include the use of small pins, small fragment compression screws or retrograde Kirschner wires. It must be remembered that whenever an osteochondral fracture has occurred, a significant ligament or capsular tear may coexist and prove to be a significant cause of subsequent morbidity (O'Donoghue, 1966).

EPIPHYSEAL FRACTURES

In children, various fractures occur which involve the growth plate (see Chapter 4). The distal femoral or proximal tibial epiphyses are partially sheared off the shafts of the respective bones, and Figure 8.7 details the various types of epiphyseal fracture (Salter and Harris, 1963). Damage to the germinal layer of the growth plate, with resultant growth arrest, is most likely with the type V fracture. However, types II–IV may also be associated with a partial growth plate arrest and children suffering from these injuries should be reviewed over a minimum of 2 years (Figures 8.8–8.12). Malunion occurs readily following the type IV fracture, and internal

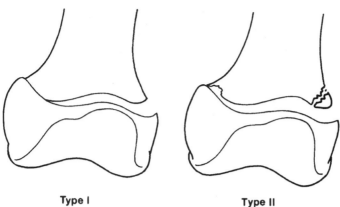

Type I   Type II

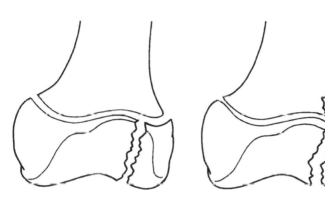

Type III   Type IV

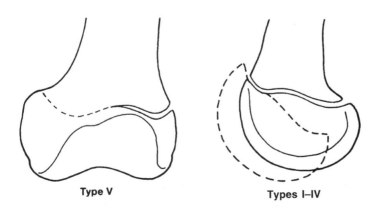

Type V   Types I–IV

Figure 8.7 *Salter–Harris (1963) classification of distal femoral epiphyseal fracture – separation. Direct injury to the perichondrial ring from an open, abrading wound may cause a partial growth arrest, which also complicates types II–V fractures in ascending order of frequency*

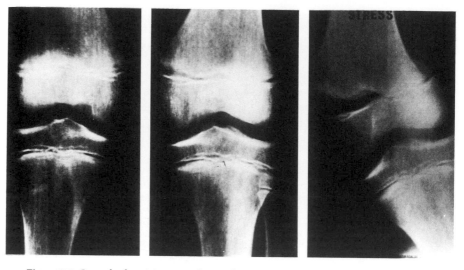

Figure 8.8 Growth plate injury may be masked

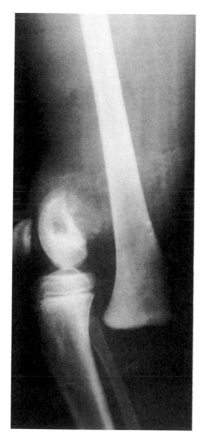

Figure 8.9 A significantly displaced type II fracture of the distal femoral epiphysis. Injury to the popliteal vessels and nerves is of principal concern

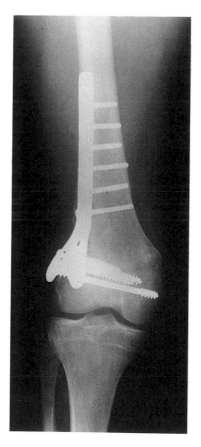

Figure 8.10 Internal fixation in the older child or adult is best ensured with a buttress plate rather than a blade plate

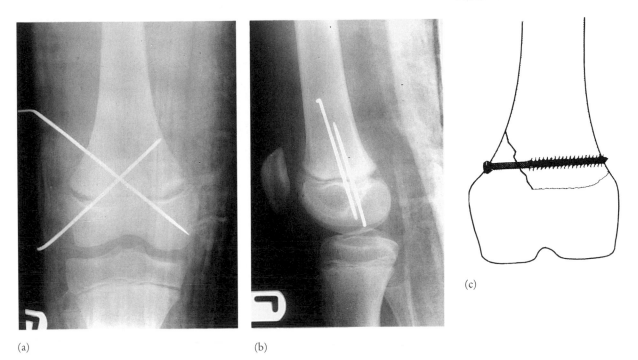

(a)   (b)

(c)

Figure 8.11 *In the younger child, reduction and fixation with Kirschner wires (a,b) or an inter-fragmentary screw (c) should be augmented with plaster cast support*

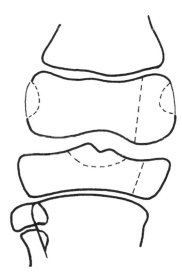

Figure 8.12 *The sites of avulsion epiphyseal fractures which merit Kirschner wire or compression screw fixation*

fixation of the types III and IV fracture is usually necessary (Macnicol, 1994). In children the tibial tuberosity may also be avulsed (Figures 8.13–8.15) and this too should be reduced and secured with a screw if there is gross displacement.

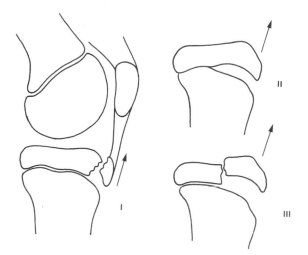

Figure 8.13 *Variations of proximal tibial epiphyseal fractures produced by the pull of the patellar tendon (separation of the whole epiphysis is rare owing to the tethering effect of the collateral ligaments and tendons). In the adult, rupture of the patellar tendon is the corresponding injury*

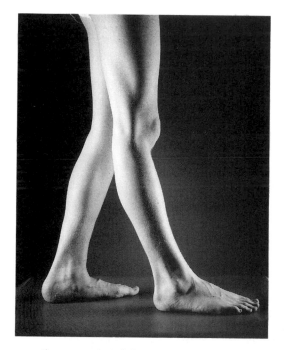

Figure 8.14 *Recurvatum (hyperextension) deformity secondary to partial growth arrest of the anterior proximal epiphyseal plate*

Loss of joint movement is less likely in children than in adults, but the principles of management remain the same, in that early movement of the knee is recommended. Cast bracing and partial weightbearing using crutches are both valuable techniques in this group of patients.

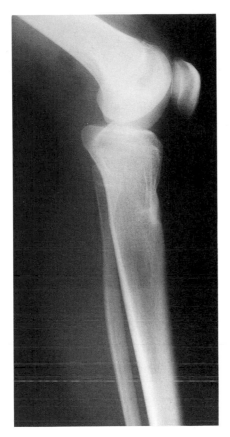

Figure 8.15 *The radiographic appearance of partial growth arrest*

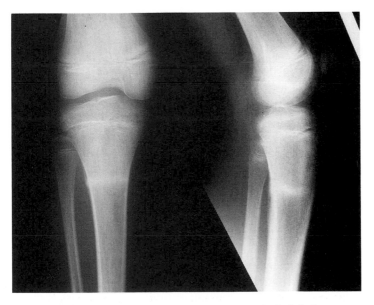

Figure 8.16 *A stress fracture of the proximal tibial shaft*

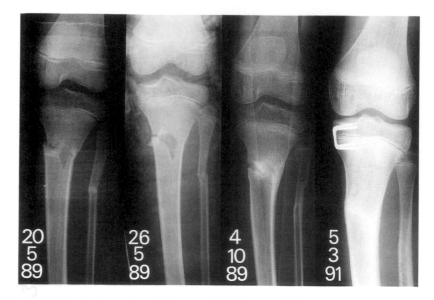

Figure 8.17 *Proximal metaphyseal fractures of the tibia may lead to a valgus malunion which does not invariably correct. Comminuted fractures of both the tibia and the fibula are most likely to angulate, and occasionally a medial stapling is required to correct the valgus deformity*

STRESS FRACTURES

Repetitive stresses to the leg may produce hairline fractures, particularly in the tibial shaft (Figure 8.16). These should be suspected in children or athletes who perform repetitive activities, whether at work or during leisure (Devas, 1963). The diagnosis can often be made by suspecting the injury and repeating a radiograph after two or three weeks. This will then show periosteal and osseous changes, and a bone scan may reveal increased blood flow at the site of the stress fracture. Occasionally these changes may be difficult to differentiate from the early stages of a bone tumour, and a careful history and follow-up is essential.

During growth a form of stress fracture occurs in relation to the attachment of tendons to bone. These 'osteochondroses' are fairly numerous throughout the skeleton, and in the region of the knee involve the tibial tuberosity (Osgood–Schlatter's disease) and the lower pole of the patella (Sinding-Larsen–Johansson syndrome). Treatment is often difficult but should include an initial period of rest, and advice and reassurance to both the child and the parents. Most of these 'growing pains' will settle at the end of skeletal growth.

Occasionally the symptoms from Osgood–Schlatter's disease may become chronic and this is said to be more common if an ossicle forms in relation to the patellar tendon distally (see Figure 4.2). Excision of this ossicle in late adolescence or early adult life may relieve symptoms, but in other respects these developmental injuries are best managed conservatively.

COMPLICATIONS OF FRACTURES

Early complications include:

- Haemarthrosis of the knee, which may merit an aspiration for the purpose of diagnosis and the relief of symptoms
- Nerve or vessel damage, which is not uncommon when a compound fracture involves the knee
- Compartment syndrome which should be relieved within 8 hours of its occurrence if permanent disability is to be avoided. This syndrome is discussed further towards the end of Chapter 9.
- Infection of a compound fracture or following surgical intervention

Late complications include:

- Chronic infection
- Malunion (Figure 8.17)
- Osteoarthritis
- Stiffness

Stiffness of the knee is a major problem after conservatively managed femoral fractures, particularly if the fracture has been significantly displaced and if movement of the knee is not encouraged at an early stage (Charnley, 1947). Stiffness is the result of both extra-articular adhesions, binding the quadriceps mechanism to the femoral shaft (Judet, 1954), and to intra-articular adhesions in certain cases. The additional factors of muscle weakness and residual deformity will also worsen any stiffness present.

Distal femoral fractures and infected injuries are far more likely to develop significant stiffness, and inappropriate internal fixation will also reduce knee movement. Usually, periosteal scar and callus reabsorb and remodel, and recovery of knee movement occurs slowly over the ensuing 18 months after injury. This progress must not be inadvisedly hastened by forced manipulation since such passive therapy may promote myositis ossificans and inhibit subsequent muscle function.

If stiffness of the knee cannot be avoided by physiotherapy throughout the period of convalescence, a quadricepsplasty may be required (Nicoll, 1963). Adhesions between the muscles and the bone must be released and the knee moved as soon as possible thereafter. The use of a commercial knee 'mobilizer' may be of great value in maintaining movement in the knee during the early postoperative period, and regular, passive movement of the knee at this stage is not particularly painful. Although distal quadricepsplasty may address the problems at the site of the fracture, there is the danger that an extension lag may persist. A proximal quadricepsplasty combined with a release of all adhesions may therefore be preferred.

More general complications which may follow any fracture of the lower limbs include deep venous thrombosis, pulmonary embolism, chest infection, malnutrition and osteoporosis. These complications are beyond the scope of this book, but will obviously influence the recovery following fractures of the knee.

References

Apley, A.G. (1956) Fracture of the lateral tibial condyle treated by skeletal traction and early mobilisation. *J. Bone Joint Surg.*, **38B**, 699–708

Burri, C., Bartzke, G., Coldewey, J. and Muggler, E. (1979) Fractures of the tibial plateau. *Clin. Orthop.*, **138**, 84–93

Charnley, J. (1947) Knee movement following fractures of the femoral shaft. *J. Bone Joint Surg.*, **29A**, 679–686

Dandy, D.J. (1992) Chondral and osteochondral lesions of the femoral condyles. In *Knee Surgery : Current Practice* (eds Aichroth, P.M. and Cannon, W.D.), Martin Dunitz, London, pp. 443–449

Devas, M.B. (1963) Stress fractures in children. *J. Bone Joint Surg.*, **45B**, 528–541

Dowd, G.E. (1982) Marginal fractures of the patella. *Injury*, **14**, 287–291

Giles, J.B., DeLee, J.C., Heckman, J.D. *et al.* Supracondylar–intercondylar fractures of the femur treated with a supracondylar plate and lag screw. *J. Bone Joint surg.*, **64A**, 864–870

Hohl, M. and Luck, J.V. (1956) Fractures of the tibial condyle. A clinical and experimental study. *J. Bone Joint Surg.*, **38A**, 1001–1018

Honkonen, S.E. and Jarvinen, M.J. (1992) Classification of fractures of the tibial condyles. *J. Bone Joint Surg.*, **74B**, 840–847

Hubbard, M.J.S. (1987) Arthroscopic surgery for chondral flaps in the knee. *J. Bone Joint Surg.*, **69B**, 794–796

Judet, R. (1954) Mobilisation of the stiff knee. *J. Bone Joint Surg.*, **41B**, 856–857

Leung, K.S., Shen, W.Y., So, W.S. *et al.* (1992) Interlocking intrameduallary nailing for supracondylar and intercondylar fractures of the distal part of the femur. *J. Bone Joint Surg.*, **73A**, 332–340

Macnicol, M.F. (1994) Indications for internal fixation. In *Children's Orthopaedics and Fractures* (eds Benson, M.K.D., Fixsen, J.A. and Macnicol, M.F.), Churchill Livingstone, Edinburgh, pp. 707–720

Müller, M.E., Allgower, M. and Willenegger, H. (1970) *Manual of Internal Fixation. Technique Recommended by the AO Group*, Springer-Verlag, Berlin

Müller, M.E., Nayeria, S. and Koch, P. (1988) *The AO Classification of Fractures*, Springer-Verlag, Berlin

Nicoll, E.A. (1963) Quadricepsplastsy. *J. Bone Joint Surg.*, **45B**, 483–490

O'Donoghue, D.H. (1966) Chondral and osteochondral fractures. *J. Trauma*, **6**, 469–481

O'Dwyer, K.J. and Bobic, V.R. (1992) Arthroscopic management of tibial plateau fractures. *Injury*, **23**, 261–264

Olerud, S. (1972) Operative treatment of supracondylar–intercondylar fractures of the femur. *J. Bone Joint surg.*, **54A**, 1015–1032

Porter, B.B. (1970) Crush fractures of the lateral tibial table *J. Bone Joint Surg.*, **52B**, 676–687

Rasmussen, P.S. and Sörensen, S.E. (1973) Tibial condylar fractures. *Injury*, **4**, 265–268

Rockwood, C.A., Green, D.P. (eds) (1991) *Fractures*, 3rd edn J. B. Lippincott, Philadelphia

Salter, R.B. and Harris, W.R. (1963) Injuries involving the epiphyseal plate. *J. Bone Joint Surg.*, **45A**, 587–592

Sanders, R., Swiontkowski, M., Rosen, H. and Helfet, D. (1991) Double-plating of comminuted, unstable fractures of the distal part of the femur. *J. Bone Joint Surg.*, **73**, 341–346

Schatzker, J., McBroom, R. and Bruce, D. (1979) The tibial plateau fracture. *Clin. Orthop.*, **138**, 94–104

Siliski, J.M., Mahsing, M. and Hofer, H.P. (1989) Supracondylar–intercondylar fractures of the femur. *J. Bone Joint Surg.*, **7A**, 95–194

Vangsness, C. Jr., DeCampos, J., Merritt, P.O. and Wiss, D.A. (1993) Meniscal injury associated with femoral shaft fractures. *J. Bone Joint Surg.*, **75B**, 207–209

9

Non-traumatic conditions

INFLAMMATORY ARTHRITIS – HAEMOPHILIA –
OSTEONECROSIS – OSTEOCHONDRITIS DISSECANS –
BLOUNT'S DISEASE – TUMOURS – COMPARTMENT
SYNDROME – DEEP VENOUS THROMBOSIS – PRESSURE
SORES

A number of 'intrinsic problems' may affect the knee and confuse the clinical assessment of the joint that is painful after presumed trauma. Quite commonly, an underlying disease process or congenital abnormality will predispose the knee to symptoms which are then precipitated by an injury, often of fairly minor degree. When considering congenital abnormalities, the following variations from normal should be remembered:

- Ligament laxity, which may be familial or in association with muscular dystrophy, Marfan's syndrome, osteogenesis imperfecta, spinal muscular atrophy, Down's syndrome and certain skeletal dysplasias
- Anomalies of the meniscus, particularly (a) the discoid lateral meniscus, and (b) cysts around the periphery or within either the lateral or medial meniscus
- Absence of one or both cruciate ligaments (sometimes in association with major skeletal abnormalities)
- Haemophilia
- Malalignment syndromes, such as persistent femoral anteversion and torsional deformities of the tibia

There are also a number of developmental conditions which may afflict the knee in the child or young adult (see Chapter 4) and these include osteochondritis dissecans, synovitis and arthropathies, metabolic diseases, tumours and infections.

Many of these problems have been discussed in other sections of the book, and this chapter will deal with inflammatory arthritis, including infection, synovial pathology, haemophilia, osteonecrosis and osteochondritis dissecans, Blount's disease and tumours. Compartment syndrome, deep venous thrombosis and pressure sores will also be described briefly insofar as they influence the function of the knee.

INFLAMMATORY ARTHRITIS

In younger patients the knee is most commonly involved if a monarticular synovitis develops, acting as a signal for the beginning of a systemic disease. It is therefore important to obtain a detailed medical history which should include questions about:

- Symptoms from inflammatory conditions of the eye, including iritis, scleritis and conjunctivitis
- Mucosal ulceration
- Respiratory and abdominal symptoms
- Urethritis
- Skin rashes
- Non-specific symptoms such as malaise, loss of weight or fevers
- A family history, with specific questioning about iritis, inflammatory bowel disease, psoriasis, gout and stiff and painful joints

Synovitis

When a synovitis develops, a minor degree of trauma may be advanced by the patient as the cause of the symptoms. A systemic condition should be suspected when the synovitic features remain or if the history is not convincingly that of trauma. A synovitis will cause the knee to feel rather doughy and warm, and may be associated with an effusion. If the skin appears reddened, then infection or a crystal synovitis should be suspected and in these instances a synovial fluid assay is diagnostic.

Synovial fluid

Synovial fluid, and tissue, if available, should be examined microscopically for the presence of pus cells and crystals (see Table 9.1). A Gram stain is sometimes recommended but usually bacteriological culture is requested and an anti-staphylococcal antibiotic is started until the causative organism is known. The culture should include media for anaerobic and tuberculous organisms in addition to standard plating. Thermography and scanning with radioisotopes may be indicated, but undoubtedly the most direct assessment is provided by arthroscopy which permits both an evaluation of the intra-articular fluid and a synovial biopsy (see Plate 40).

Certain blood tests are of value, but may not necessarily provide more than a clue to the diagnosis. The ESR is often raised, but is a non-specific test. The white blood cell and C-reactive protein are elevated. The rheumatoid factor, representing the production of a macro-immunoglobulin against IgG, may be negative in the majority of cases with juvenile chronic arthritis in childhood and in 30% of adults with rheumatoid arthritis. Tests for the serum uric acid and titres against staphylococcus and streptococcus may be helpful, and an anti-streptococcal titre consistently below 200 units makes rheumatic fever unlikely. The HLA B27 antigen is positive in 5–10% of the normal population, but may be a useful pointer in a patient with ankylosing spondylitis, Reiter's syndrome or with an arthritis that is associated with inflammatory bowel disease.

Table 9.1 Synovial fluid analysis as an aid to diagnosis

Blood	Fracture, ligament rupture, synovial tear (haemophilia, haemangioma)
Fat	Osteochondral fracture, fat-pad lesion
Debris	Articular cartilage damage including chondromalacia, meniscal tear
Cells	(a) Monocyte predominance in osteoarthritis
	(b) Polymorphonuclear cell predominance in inflammatory synovitis including rheumatoid arthritis and septic arthritis
Crystals	(a) Gout (urate) – feathery crystals
	(b) Pseudogout (monophosphate) – rectangular crystals
Lactate, acidity and lysosomal enzymes	Increased in inflammatory conditions
Lysosomal enzymes	Increased in painful synovitis
Complement	(a) Increased in Reiter's syndrome and gout
	(b) Increased in osteoarthritis
	(c) Decreased in rheumatoid arthritis

Synovial biopsy

Arthroscopic examination will not only allow an accurate sampling of the inflamed synovium, but will also help to rule out the following mechanical lesions that may cause a synovitis:

- Meniscus tear
- Loose body
- Articular cartilage abnormality
- Plica/impingement
- Fracture

Synovial biopsy, although a very direct test, can again only indicate the presence of an inflammatory condition; the following histological changes may be observed:

- Hypertrophy of the synovial fronds
- Proliferation of the superficial synovial cells
- A chronic inflammatory cell infiltrate, occasionally with the development of lymphoid follicles
- Cell necrosis in patches of the synovial tissue
- Deposition of fibrin both within and on the surface of the synovium

The synovial biopsy will aid in diagnosing gout and pseudogout (crystal synovitis), pigmented villonodular synovitis, sarcoidosis, synovial chondromatosis (Figure 9.1a,b), malignant synovioma, and specific infections including tuberculosis.

Treatment

If an inflammatory arthritis is considered to be present, a number of relatively conservative measures can be used to lessen symptoms and

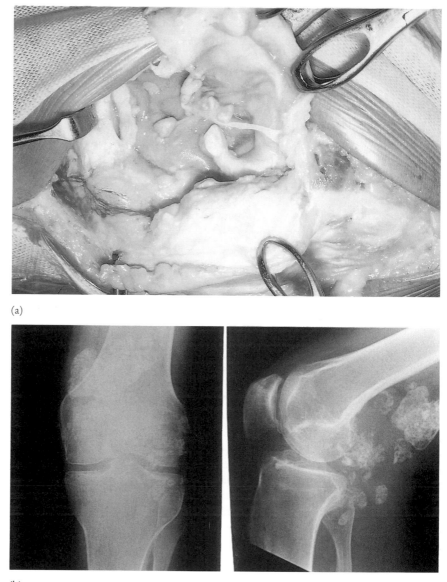

(a)

(b)

Figure 9.1 *Arthrotomy reveals craggy irregularities (a) of the synovial membrane affected by synovial chondromatosis (b)*

preserve function in the joint. Splintage may be of value in the early stages, when the inflammation is poorly controlled, but prolonged immobilization will lead to disuse atrophy of muscle and stiffness. Hence, a balanced approach must be ensured, with preservation of muscle bulk by means of isometric exercises, and the subsequent maintenance of a functional arc of movement by controlled and carefully directed physiotherapy.

Ice packs may lessen pain from muscle spasm, and mild heat in the form of hydrotherapy or wax baths may permit a greater degree of function in

Table 9.2 Anti-inflammatory analgesic drugs

Simple analgesics	Low doses of aspirin (acetyl salicylic acid)
	Benoral (benorylate)
	Panadol (paracetamol)
	Codeine phosphate
	DF 118 (dihydrocodeine tartrate)
Non-steroidal anti-inflammatory agents	Weaker preparations:
	Brufen (ibuprofen)
	Naprosyn (naproxen)
	Fenopron (fenoprofen)
	Clinoril (sulindac)
	Feldene (piroxicam)
	Rheumox (azapropazone)
	Voltarol (diclofenac sodium)
	Ponstan (mefenamic acid)
	Stronger preparations:
	Full doses of aspirin (acetyl salicylic acid)
	Indocid (indomethacin)
Local corticosteroid injections	
	Depomedrone (methylprednisolone acetate)
	Hydrocortisone acetate
	Adcortyl (triamcinolone acetonide)

the joint. Unfortunately, the benefits from these techniques are short lived and some other means of reducing the synovitis is usually necessary. In this context, radiant heat, including short-wave diathermy, may markedly worsen symptoms, as will over-vigorous physiotherapy.

Anti-inflammatory analgesia is usually beneficial, although no one drug will remain effective indefinitely, and various patients will react in different ways to the different preparations. A policy of monitoring symptoms and alternating the drug treatments is therefore advisable.

Table 9.2 lists the various forms of anti-inflammatory analgesic agents that can be used. These drugs are unsafe if combined with oral anti-coagulants, hypoglycaemic agents and other highly protein-bound compounds. Gastrointestinal bleeding may also be produced. Various enteric-coated drugs are therefore available, and analgesics may also be given in suppository form.

Synovectomy

If the synovitis fails to respond to these measures, a synovectomy may be necessary and still finds a place in the treatment of the patient with rheumatoid arthritis and the younger haemophiliac. A subtotal synovectomy is quite possible surgically, but must be offered in good time, before the articular cartilage has been extensively affected. There is always a risk that the range of movement will lessen owing to the postoperative scarring, and the principal indication for synovectomy is unremitting pain, particularly if the range of movement is lessening rapidly.

Subtotal synovectomy is now possible arthroscopically using a motorized shaver. Rehabilitation is usually more rapid than after open synovectomy, but great care must be taken with the placement of portals and protection of the articular surfaces. Medical synovectomy using radioactive gold or yttrium 90 may be more appropriate in older patients or in cases of recurrent symptoms.

Septic arthritis

The knee is the most common site of sepsis in later childhood and adult life. In the pre-school child, and especially in infancy, the hip is the prime target joint, partly because the femoral metaphysis is intra-articular so that infection readily spreads from a proximal femoral osteomyelitis. Multifocal septic arthritis should always be suspected in the septicaemic patient, particularly if the host is known to be immunocompromised.

Irrigation of the joint is considered to be of value, and the combination of antibiotic treatment and lavage prevents collagen destruction more effectively than antibiotics and aspiration alone (Daniel *et al.*, 1976). Nevertheless, the biochemical effects of the irrigant may also be deleterious, and therefore Ringer's lactate is preferred to other solutions and should neither be chilled nor used in excessive volume.

The differential diagnosis includes the various arthropathies of childhood, whether seronegative or seropositive, synovitis in association with rheumatic fever and the exanthemata, and neoplastic conditions of the synovium and skeleton (see pages172–176). Delay in diagnosis and inadequate decompression remain the critical factors (Goldenberg *et al.*, 1975) and a series of recent papers has confirmed the value of the arthroscope (Ivey and Clark, 1985; Skyhar and Mubarak, 1987; Stanitski *et al.*, 1989; Ohl *et al.*, 1991). This form of treatment is superior to aspiration where approximately one in three cases will be left with residual necrotic and fibrinous debris and adhesion formation. The smaller diameter (3.8 mm rather than 5 mm) arthroscope may be indicated in pre-school children, but the larger sheath is more effective and will allow a cannula to be inserted in the joint for intermittent lavage. Every 8 hours for two or three days 10 ml of Ringer's lactate can be instilled, combined with marcaine and morphine if pain is severe. Antibiotic should be given intravenously, and the potentially harmful effects of concentrated antibiotic upon articular cartilage mean that concentrated drug solutions should not be inserted in the joint.

A general anaesthetic is recommended rather than local anaesthesia when arthroscopy is being considered for the child (see Figure 3.5), although Jarrett *et al.* (1981) found that regional or local block was satisfactory in adults. The essence of arthroscopic treatment is that it should ensure complete decompression of the joint, with the breakdown of adhesions and loculations using a blunt trocar, and that all recesses of the cavity should be thoroughly irrigated with a non-irritant fluid. Even if a cannula is left *in situ* to allow intermittent lavage, the use of continuous passive motion and early active movement should be encouraged. Reaccumulation of pus and the return of pain should be dealt with by further irrigation and by repeat arthroscopy if necessary. In the early case this approach will ensure a satisfactory functional recovery with minimal postoperative morbidity. In the chronic or recurrent case the outcome is less certain and residual stiffness and articular cartilage damage are likely to persist.

The range of organisms cultured from the infected knee does not differ from that seen in other large joints, particularly the hip. Staphylococcal organisms are the most likely, but streptococcal, Gram-negative and anaerobic organisms must also be suspected, sometimes in combination:

Staphylococcus aureus
Staph. epidermidis
Streptococcus pyogenes
Haemophilus influenza
Strep. pneumoniae
Pseudomonas aeruginosa
Strep. faecalis
Escherichia coli
Proteus spp., *Klebsiella* spp., *Salmonella* spp.
Anaerobic organisms (rare)

Immune deficiency is less common after the neonatal period (Macnicol, 1986), but may play a part in the indolent septic arthritis encountered in older, arthritic patients and in those suffering from a polyarthropathy. The antibiotic of choice will depend on sensitivity patterns, and should commence with the intravenous administration of a 'best guess' agent, such as flucloxacillin and augmentin, followed by alternative drugs as indicated. The antibiotic therapy which follows is dependent on hospital policy and subsequent cultures:

Flucloxacillin
Gentamicin
Clindamycin
Fusidic acid
Cefuroxime
Cefotaxime
Co-trimoxazole
Ampicillin

Ohl *et al.* (1991) reported a 10-month follow-up of 16 septic knees in children, with good early results following early weightbearing after arthroscopic debridement. However, the long-term results following infection are poorly recorded and some permanent articular cartilage loss is inevitable after late treatment. Extensive surgery may be required to correct late deformity if the growth plate has been involved (Figures 9.2 and 9.3a,b).

Synovial conditions

Haemangioma of the fat-pad (see Plate 46) produces episodes of haemarthrosis and locking, eventually leading to loss of movement if the bleeds go unchecked (Paley and Jackson, 1986; Juhl and Krebs, 1989). Stimulus of the growth plate may result in slight overgrowth of the limb. Arthroscopic treatment is effective, as it may also be in haemophilia (Klein *et al.*, 1987; Limbird and Dennis, 1987).

Synovial chondromatosis (Carey, 1983; Coolican and Dandy, 1989; Kistler, 1991) is a rare but recognized acquired condition in childhood (see Plate 48). Pain, swelling, catching and locking are again the features, which

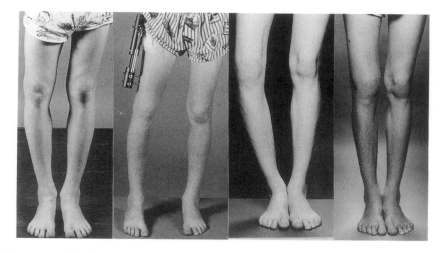

Figure 9.2 *Infantile septic arthritis of the right knee producing distal femoral growth arrest (shortening and varus)*

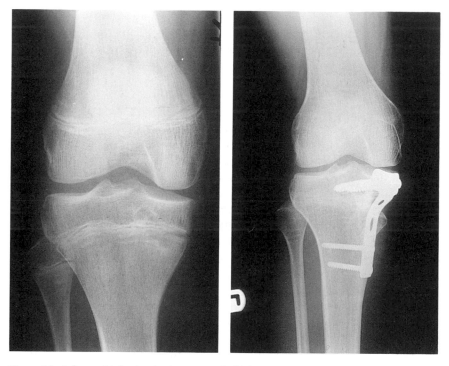

Figure 9.3 *A focus of infection in the proximal tibial growth plate (a), producing varus deformity which required correction by a later osteotomy (b)*

may also characterize torsion of a synovial polyp, pigmented villonodular synovitis (Giron *et al.*, 1991) and synovioma.

A generalized synovitis is pathognomonic of juvenile chronic arthritis but may also be seen in mild haemophilia, in Lyme disease (Schoen *et al.*, 1991) and after viral illnesses. Skin conditions such as eczema and psoriasis also seem to predispose the younger patient to knee effusions.

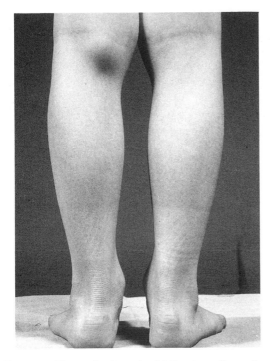

Figure 9.4 The popliteal cyst in childhood usually resolves

The plica syndrome generated much interest a decade ago but is now accepted as one of a number of causes of anterior knee pain. When a thickened band can be palpated as it rolls or clicks over the medial femoral condyle, the diagnosis can be sustained, particularly when abrasion is present over the articular edge of the condyle. Excision of the thickened band or shelf of synovium is often effective (Koshino and Okamoto, 1985; Patel, 1986) but the interior of the knee must be thoroughly inspected for other pathology at the time of arthroscopy and extra-articular lesions should always be considered by appropriate preoperative examination and investigations (Joyce and Mankin, 1983).

A popliteal cyst commonly presents in mid-childhood (Figure 9.4) without the knowledge of the patient but to the parents' alarm. The swelling is usually a semimembranosus bursa which communicates with the knee joint but is not a pathological process. Histology of the wall of the cyst reveals a non-specific inflammatory reaction, with a fibrotic response proportional to the chronicity of the lesion. Radiography is advisable in order to rule out skeletal changes, but ultrasound, arthrographic and magnetic resonance assessment are rarely indicated.

In childhood the cyst usually disappears and its excision is quite unnecessary. Aspiration is appropriate if the knee appears synovitic, but this will only aid in diagnosis and is not therapeutic. In older patients a popliteal cyst develops as a manifestation of repeated effusions in the knee. In association with osteoarthritis the term 'Baker's cyst' is often used. Excision of a large cyst may be indicated if the symptoms are severe, but recurrence is likely if the primary inflammatory process is not addressed. The injection of local steroid preparations after aspiration of the cyst is therefore preferable, at least initially.

Rupture of a Baker's cyst may produce symptoms which mimic a deep venous thrombosis in the calf. Arthrographic or MR imaging are diagnostic and the condition is treated symptomatically with supportive stockings, physiotherapy to maintain power and knee motion, and short-term anti-inflammatory analgesia.

HAEMOPHILIA

Haemophilia is a genetically-determined coagulation disorder which occurs predominantly in males (types A and B) with an incidence of approximately 1 in 8000. Haemophilia C (von Willebrand's disease) affects both men and women, the female being an asymptomatic carrier of the sex-linked recessive gene. Haemophilia A is caused by a deficiency of factor VIII (anti-haemophilic factor: AHF) and constitutes 80% of all cases. Haemophilia B (Christmas disease) results from a deficiency of factor IX (Christmas factor or plasma thromboplastin component).

The general clinical manifestations of haemophilia include a tendency to bleed readily from lacerations and mucosal surfaces. Haemarthroses are common, causing pain, distension and warmth of the joint (see Plate 47). Typically, a haemophiliac patient will feel that there is a bleed within a joint before the clinical signs become evident. Haematomata and haemophilic cysts may develop in the thigh, buttock, abdomen, calf and hand. The cysts are either simple, contained within muscle fascia, or deeper, in which case they may be either juxtacortical, between muscle attachment and bone, or subperiosteal, which is the most common site.

Pathology

After a haemarthrosis has developed in the knee, there is a subsequent release of haemosiderin as blood corpuscles break down. This irritant material in relatively large dosage produces a synovial haemosiderosis. An initial low-grade synovitis eventually becomes fulminating, and as severe as any rheumatoid arthritis. Worse still, the synovial haemosiderosis predisposes the joint to further bleeds.

In time the synovitis progresses to a fibrotic stage, producing contracture of the capsule. The articular cartilage becomes eroded by lysosomal enzymes, released from the inflamed synovium which grows across the joint as a pannus (Figure 9.5). The chondrocytes perish from an excess of iron pigment, and an associated pressure necrosis.

The knee joint is involved in at least 50% of all patients with haemophilic arthropathy and the presentation clinically may be either acute, subacute or chronic. Occasionally, the patient is unaware of having a particular bleeding tendency, but recurrent haemarthroses in a joint such as the knee should alert the clinician to this possibility. Spontaneous bleeding may also occur from localized haemangiomas within the knee, but are rarely as troublesome as the recurrent haemarthroses of the severe haemophiliac.

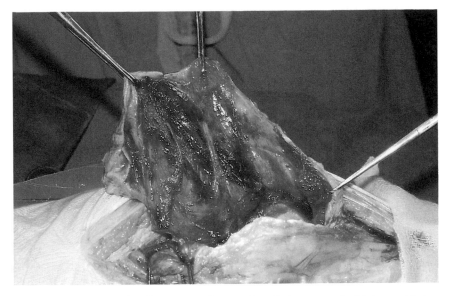

Figure 9.5 In haemophilia, the synovium becomes heavily impregnated with haemosiderin

Radiography

The radiographic features of a knee affected by haemophilic arthropathy include soft-tissue swelling, epiphyseal overgrowth (Figure 9.6) osteoporosis and thickening of the haemosiderotic synovium. Cysts and subchondral sclerosis develop around the margins of the knee joint in the more chronic cases and eventually the standard osteoarthritic changes of narrowing of the

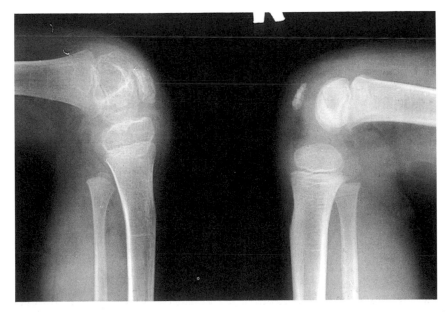

Figure 9.6 Epiphyseal overgrowth and soft-tissue thickening as a result of repeated haemarthroses. Note the Harris growth arrest lines

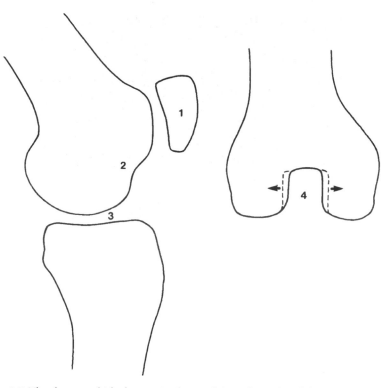

Figure 9.7 *The changes which characterize haemophilic arthropathy of the knee (1, 'squaring' of the patella; 2, notching of the femoral condyle; 3, narrowing and sclerosis of the joint; 4, widening of the femoral intercondylar notch)*

joint space, increasing sclerosis and deformity occur. Petterson *et al.* (1980) developed a grading system, scoring from 0–13, based upon these radiographic changes. The progression of the arthropathy can therefore be described and applied to reviews of therapy.

A characteristic squaring of the patella is seen, and in association with this the intercondylar femoral notch becomes deepened and widened (Figure 9.7). The femoral condyles may become indented by impaction of the anterior tibial articular surface, and this is hastened by the fact that the tibia gradually subluxes posteriorly and externally (Figure 9.8). A flexion deformity therefore becomes irreversible, not only because of the fibrotic component, but as a result of impingement between the tibia and femur.

Treatment

Treatment should embrace two principles:

- Prevention of haemorrhages by prompt treatment with factor VIII prophylaxis
- Preservation of a useful arc of knee movement

Factor VIII or IX is given by intravenous infusion in order to produce normal concentrations in the circulation. The knee should be immobilized in a backshell, which can be readily fashioned in polypropylene, and

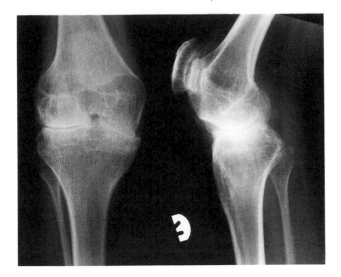

Figure 9.8 *Gross radiographic changes of haemophilic arthropathy include posterior subluxation of the tibia and an irreversible flexion deformity*

compression is applied by circumferential elasticated bandaging. Aspiration of the joint should be avoided; instead, static quadriceps exercises are instructed in order to increase intra-articular pressure. By this means the swelling should decrease progressively over 1–2 weeks. Extension should be preserved as fully as possible by ensuring quadriceps muscle tone, and thereafter flexion is regained by hamstring drill. The team approach is essential, combining the skills of the physician, orthopaedic surgeon, physiotherapist, general practitioner, specialist nurse and social worker.

In cases where a chronic synovitis has developed but the joint surfaces are still relatively well preserved, a case can be made for surgical synovectomy. This is necessarily subtotal, but will reduce the incidence of subsequent haemorrhage, although possibly at the expense of movement since fibrosis is produced by the surgery. Therefore patellofemoral mobility and knee extension must be ensured. Limbird and Dennis (1987) recommend the use of continuous passive motion after synovectomy, combined with full factor VIII cover. Arthroscopic intervention early in the course of the disease may help to control haemorrhage from localized sites in the knee and the morbidity is thereby much reduced (Weidel, 1990). Effective prophylaxis with heat-treated or recombinant factor VIII, preferably by educating the patients to the benefits of home therapy, has also reduced the severe disability that used to result from a progressive haemophilic arthropathy. Ultrasound, and CT and MR scanning reveal early articular and synovial changes before they become apparent on X-ray, and will also define subchondral and soft-tissue cysts.

In association with appropriate physiotherapy, to improve all components of the quadriceps group, the use of posterior splints and wedging casts is of value, and there may be a place for 'reverse dynamic slings', which distract and gradually extend the flexed joint. However, in cases where tibiofemoral impingement is occurring anteriorly, such measures are

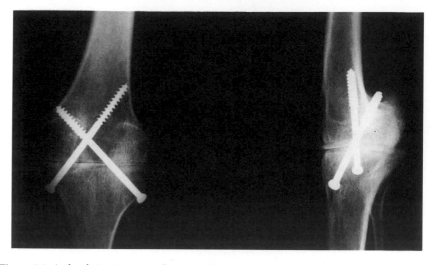

Figure 9.9 *Arthrodesis using crossed compression screws*

doomed to fail and may promote further haemorrhage within the joint. In these cases, particularly if pain is troublesome and haemarthroses recurrent, a total joint replacement or arthrodesis (Figure 9.9) may have to be considered. Surgery may also be required if a muscle haematoma or cyst develops.

OSTEONECROSIS

Osteonecrosis affects the older patient but may occasionally be seen in younger individuals with Gaucher's disease, systemic lupus erythematosus and rheumatoid-related conditions. Sickle cell disease and other haemoglobinopathies may also precipitate a problem, as may irradiation. Corticosteroid therapy for autoimmune disease or following renal transplantation, and in conditions such as severe asthma or the lymphomas, accounts for most of the drug-related cases, and the association with alcoholism, and with Caisson disease, is well established. The position and size of the lesion is prognostically significant, as are the alignment of the limb and the speed of enlargement. Involvement of more than half the medial femoral condyle in the varus knee inevitably leads to osteoarthritis and disabling pain.

Ahlbäck *et al.* (1968) are credited with the first recognition of the idiopathic form which progresses from the stage of normal radiographs to slight flattening of the weightbearing segment, as in Perthes' disease. At this stage radioisotope bone scanning and MR imaging will define the extent of the lesion accurately. A radiolucent area gradually becomes apparent, surrounded by a sclerotic halo (Motohashi *et al.*, 1991). As the subchondral plate collapses and deforms, the affected femorotibial compartment becomes increasingly irregular and arthritic.

Treatment of the early lesion includes protected weightbearing, thigh exercises and anti-inflammatory agents. Surgical intervention is based upon the merits of each case, aided by the use of arthroscopy. Core decompression (Jacobs *et al.*, 1989), tibial osteotomy (Koshino, 1982), allografts and knee replacement have a place in treatment.

OSTEOCHONDRITIS DISSECANS

Paré first described loose bodies of the knee in 1558, and Paget (1870) considered that they resulted from avascular separation, the so-called 'quiet necrosis'. The osteochondritic change in childhood is relatively benign, the juvenile form representing an alteration in distal femoral ossification rather than a progressive lesion. Males are twice as commonly affected and trauma is often implicated.

An ischaemic necrosis of the bone seems unlikely since there are no end-arteries in the distal femur, which is the usual site of osteochondritis dissecans (Figures 9.10 and 9.11a,b); furthermore, histological examination infrequently shows cellular necrosis. In this sense, osteochondritis dissecans should be distinguished from the other forms of osteochondritis (the osteochondroses) where there is a definite loss of blood supply. Although a positive family history may be recorded, the hereditary evidence is conflicting and usually the condition appears sporadically.

It seems most likely that in the teenager and adult, trauma may have a significant part to play in the development of the lesion, possibly in as many as 50% of the cases reported. Perhaps the injury produced a stress fracture but it is not known whether the trauma is exogenous, in which case very major forces have to be applied to the knee, or is endogenous, as a result

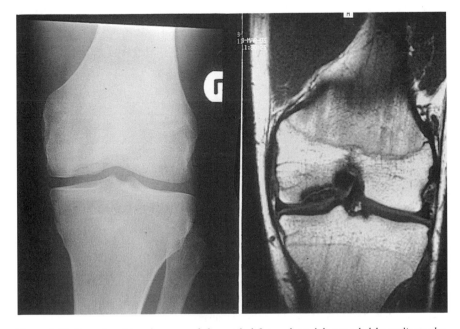

Figure 9.10 *Osteochondritis dissecans of the medial femoral condyle revealed by radiography and a magnetic resonance scan*

(a)

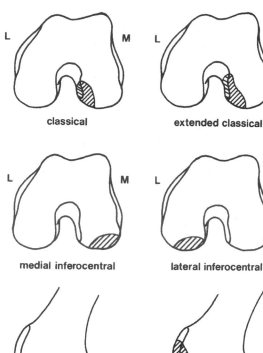

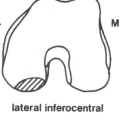

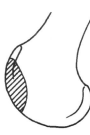

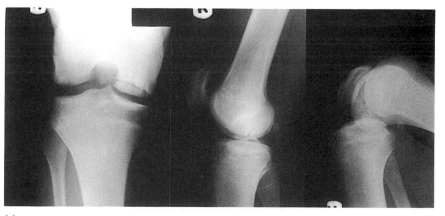

(a)

Figure 9.11 (a) *Sites of osteochondritis dissecans (After Aichroth, 1971). (b) A large medial inferocentral separation*

of regular impaction against the femoral condyle by a prominent tibial spine, a discoid lateral meniscus or a subluxing patella. The healing capacity of the osteochondritic fragment is very variable, but is poor if the true 'dissecans' or separated form is present.

Both the juvenile and adult lesions should be distinguished from a true, acute osteochondral fracture, which separates from a bed of bleeding cancellous bone (see Plates 41 and 42). The osteochondritic fragment, in contrast, is covered with fibrous tissue or hyperplastic cartilage, and is associated with an effusion, but not with a haemarthrosis since the defect is relatively avascular.

Sites where osteochondritis dissecans may be encountered radiographically are shown in Figure 9.11 and the condition may be bilateral in up to a quarter of cases. A loose body is found in between a third and a half of all knees, and males are affected twice as commonly as females. There may be a correlation with genu recurvatum, valgus or varus deformity of the knee and patellar subluxation, and an association with anomalies such as discoid lateral meniscus and epiphyseal dysplasia has been described.

The classic site is at the lateral aspect of the medial femoral condyle, and it is now believed that the prognosis is better in these cases (Twyman *et al.*, 1991; Garrett, 1991). The lateral femoral condyle is affected in some 20% of cases (Aichroth, 1971), and rarely the process affects the femoral sulcus (Smith, 1990) or the patella (Edwards and Bentley, 1977).

Constitutional factors are of importance, with a positive family history in some patients and the association with discoid lateral meniscus in others. Symptoms are relatively non-specific: aching pain, locking or clicking, recurrent effusions and limp. Wilson's sign (Wilson, 1967) is based upon the fact that the tibial spines may impinge against the femoral condyle when the tibia is internally rotated with the knee extended, and tapping over the femoral condyle (See Plate 5a,b) elicits tenderness compared to the rest of the knee.

Management

Evaluation requires four radiographic views of the knee augmented by tomography, isotope bone scanning, CT scanning and MR scans as necessary. Monitoring is best achieved by isotope scanning or the MR scan, whereas staging the lesion (Figure 9.12) relies upon arthroscopy. If the area

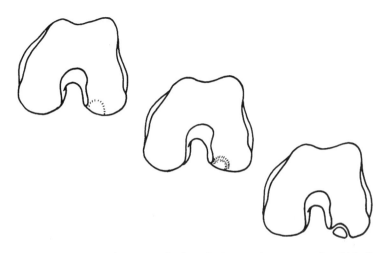

Figure 9.12 Stages in the formation of a loose body secondary to osteochondritis dissecans

is demarcated by softened hyaline cartilage but there is no breach in its surface, a conservative approach is indicated, particularly in patients before skeletal maturity. Athletic activities should be restricted, but there is no benefit from immobilization or non-weightbearing.

Arthroscopic drilling of the lesion may relieve the symptoms and is considered to hasten healing (Bradley and Dandy, 1989), although there are no controlled trials to confirm this. Drilling attempts to traumatize the base of the fragment without undue articular cartilage injury. Both retrograde and reversed drilling have been promoted, each technique purporting to bring in fresh blood supply and possibly cells to the line of cleavage. Removal of a hinging fragment, curettage of the base and fixation is acceptable if the lesion is large and reasonably congruent. Excision should only be considered with small or fragmented lesions, particularly away from the weightbearing surface of the condyle, or if the fragment cannot be reduced anatomically. The depth of the bone base can be increased to accommodate the lesion which should never be left proud of the joint surface.

Smillie (1957) used pins or screws to stabilize the lesion, and fixation with K wires was felt to produce better results than excision by Hughston *et al.* (1984). Herbert screw fixation for smaller fragments (Thomson, 1987) and countersunk small fragment AO compression screws are now established as effective implants. When operating arthroscopically a small cannula should be used to prevent the guide wire from breaking, and a cannulated screw system should be used. The implant must be accurately positioned, using two screws for larger fragments, and the knee monitored for 6 months postoperatively to check the position of the screw as well as the appearances of the lesion. Bone pins (Lindholm and Pylkkänen, 1974) and absorbable pins (Orthosorb, Johnson and Johnson) have yet to prove themselves as safe and effective options, and the use of fibrin glue (Tussucol) is still experimental. Osteochondral allografting (Garrett, 1991) may be appropriate when facilities permit but, when possible, the separated lesion should be replaced in preference. The primary problem of patellar instability should additionally be dealt with if it coexists with the rare condition of patellar osteochondritis dissecans (Pfeiffer *et al.*, 1991) (see Figure 7.17). Bradley and Dandy (1989) have questioned whether true osteochondritis dissecans ever appears at sites other than the classic site (Figures 9.11 and 9.12) and consider that distal femoral ossification patterns (Caffey *et al.*, 1958) are unrelated to the condition.

BLOUNT'S DISEASE (TIBIA VARA)

In rare instances the normal bow-leg deformity of a toddler fails to correct (Figure 9.13a–c; see also Plate 26) and the medial tibial growth plate collapses rather than being stimulated under compression. Blount (1937) described the progressive varus and internal rotation deformity of the upper tibia, noting that the medial proximal metaphysis became fragmented and then beaked (Figure 9.14). Undiagnosed trauma or infection may cause the unilateral adolescent form, but the classical bilateral condition is developmental and poorly understood (Greene, 1993).

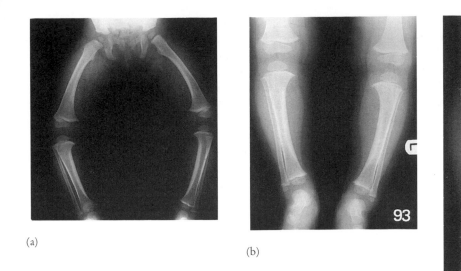

(a)

(b)

(c)

Figure 9.13(a–c) Genu varum in early childhood usually corrects (see also Plate 26)

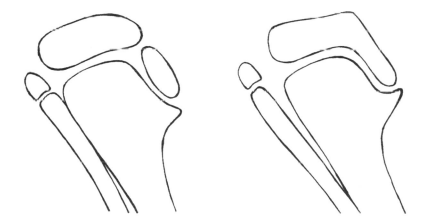

Figure 9.14 The stages of Blount's disease producing a teeter deformity of the proximal tibia

In the toddler it is customary to observe the child with serial measurements and radiographs over a period of 2–3 years. Bracing is difficult to apply for prolonged periods and is poorly tolerated by the child. Therefore by the age of 4–6 a proximal tibial valgus osteotomy is advised, in order to correct the internal rotation and to produce 5–10° of valgus (Langenskiöld, 1981).

If a medial growth plate tether develops between the ages of 8 and 10 years, it should be excised and the site of the resected bony bar filled with fat, Silastic or dental cement. Osteotomy alone at this age is unlikely to succeed, but may be combined with excision of the bar. Tomography or CT scanning will define the size of the bar and external fixation, with distraction using the Iliazarov frame, is tolerated by the older child.

As the child nears adolescence, the proximal tibial surface may be severely tented. Function is further impaired by the presence of ligament laxity, which allows a coronal rocking movement. The medial tibial plateau may then require elevation and support (Siffert, 1982) using bone graft or an excised segment of fibula. Lateral proximal tibial epiphysiodesis is combined with this reconstruction if the child has 2 or more years (over 1 cm) of longitudinal growth at that site. In unilateral cases, a contralateral proximal tibial epiphysiodesis will control the leg-length discrepancy which complicates the condition.

TUMOURS

Soft-tissue swellings

The knee joint may be the site of a neoplastic growth, either in the soft tissues or in bone. Any anatomical structure forming part of the knee can enlarge abnormally. Thus fat may produce a lipoma, and fibrous tissue a sarcomatous tumour, including fibrosarcoma or a neurofibroma if there is a neural element in the tissues. Tumours of muscle (leiomyoma, leiomyosarcoma and rhabdomyoscarcoma), vascular tumours, such as angiomata (see Plate 46) and various forms of angiosarcoma (haemangioendotheliomas and haemangiopericytomas) and several fibromatous conditions within bone as well as in the surrounding tissue will produce lumps around the knee, although they are rare. These have to be distinguished from the more common proliferative inflammatory lesions such as pigmented villonodular synovitis and bursitis. Synovioma is a relatively rare but malignant tumour of the synovial lining; aggressive treatment is required in the form of radical excision.

Cystic lumps around the knee (see Plates 29–31) generally develop insidiously, whereas trauma may produce more rapid swellings, such as a haematoma, arteriovenous fistula or abnormalities in the contour of the muscle as a result of rupture or avulsion from a bony origin. Infective conditions may result in abscesses and enlargement of soft tissue, and in chronic inflammatory conditions such as gout and rheumatoid arthritis, tophi and rheumatoid nodules are produced, respectively, and may present over the extensor surface of the knee.

Bone tumours

Bone tumours involving the distal femur and proximal tibia are relatively common, and account for between 20% and 25% of all skeletal primary neoplasias. Gerhardt *et al.* (1990) reviewed 199 cases of neoplasia affecting the knee in childhood, noting that the lesions were referred more commonly in the older child. Benign tumours accounted for half the cases, and in decreasing order of frequency were osteochondroma, non-ossifying fibroma, chondroblastoma, osteoid osteoma, aneurysmal bone cyst, giant cell tumour, chondromyxoid fibroma, simple bone cyst and fibrous dysplasia. Benign lesions tend to be small and well marginated, with minimal or no cortical alteration and no soft-tissue mass adjoining them. Benign latent

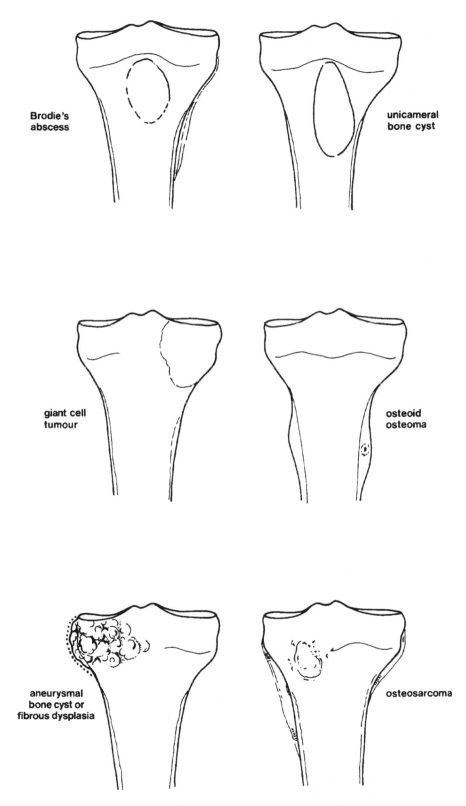

Figure 9.15 Radiographic features of the more common lesions affecting the proximal tibia

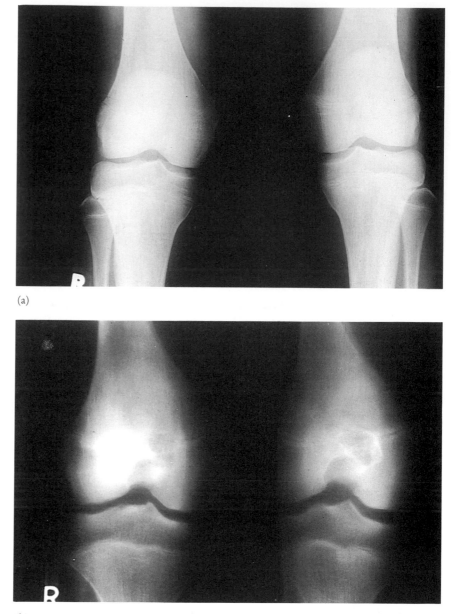

(a)

(b)

Figure 9.16 *Chondroblastoma of the distal femur (a), only apparent on tomography (b)*

tumours such as fibrous cortical defect or dysplasia should be differentiated from active lesions, for example aneurysmal bone cyst or chondroblastoma (Lodwick *et al.*, 1980).

Radiographically, these lesions produce slightly different appearances, as
shown in Figure 9.15, but quite often the diagnosis cannot be made with
certainty and a histological examination is essential. Non-ossifying fibroma,
or fibrous cortical defect, is very common in the end of a long bone during

growth, and these are rarely of any concern. Other benign tumours encountered in the younger patient, including chondromyxoid fibroma, fibrous dysplasia, benign chondroblastoma (see Figures 9.16a,b) and diaphyseal aclasis may give cause for concern and therefore merit follow-up.

Investigation of malignant tumour includes:

- Computerized tomography
- Magnetic resonance imaging
- Angiography
- Soft-tissue and bone biopsy

As with soft-tissue tumours, the cell of origin of bone tumours can usually be defined and hence the following classification is of some histological value.

Osteogenic
1 Osteoid osteoma
2 Osteochondroma
    (a) Single: sessile or pedunculated
    (b) Multiple
3 Osteosarcoma
4 Parosteal sarcoma

Chondrogenic
1 Chondroma (or enchondroma)
2 Benign chondroblastoma
3 Chondromyxoid fibroma

Fibrogenic
1 Non-osteogenic fibroma
2 Fibrous dysplasia
3 Fibrosarcoma
4 Malignant fibrous histiocytoma

Bone 'cyst'
1 Unicameral
2 Aneurysmal
3 Giant cell tumour
4 Ewing's sarcoma
5 Brown tumour of hyperparathyroidism
6 Metastasis from other site

The treatment of these bone tumours is beyond the scope of this book, but they should be recognized in the differential diagnosis of the painful knee, and always suspected in cases where the history is non-specific or where there is progressive swelling and tenderness of the femur or tibia.

Many benign tumours will heal or remain asymptomatic, and treatment is only directed to those that become symptomatic, usually because of an incipient stress fracture, enlargement (Figures 9.17a–c and 9.18) or developing malignancy. The sarcomas of bone can sometimes be treated by radical resection and chemotherapy, thus saving the leg. All too often, however, the only surgical recourse is segmental resection, an upper thigh amputation or hip disarticulation.

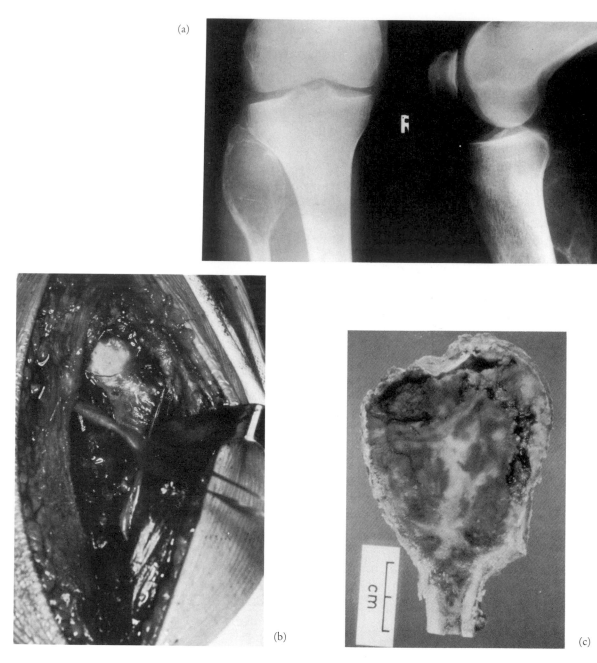

Figure 9.17(a–c) A giant cell tumour of the proximal fibula

COMPARTMENT SYNDROME

Exercise-induced compartment syndrome

The muscle compartments of the calf are shown in Figure 9.19. Those that commonly affect the athlete are the anterior compartment and the deep posterior compartment. After 10–20 minutes of strenuous exertion, pressure can be shown to rise within the anterolateral compartment, from a normal

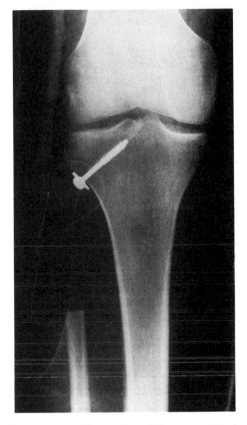

Figure 9.18 *Radiographic appearances after excision of the tumour. The lateral (fibular) collateral ligament and biceps tendon have been reattached to the proximal tibia*

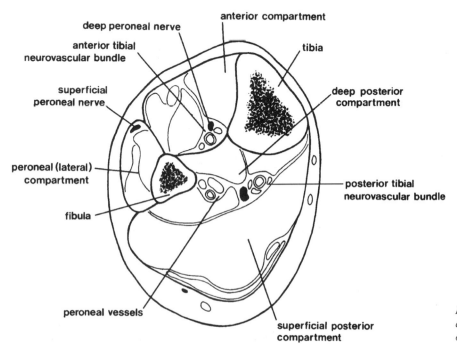

Figure 9.19 *Cross-section of the calf to show the fascial boundaries of the compartments*

resting level of approximately 4 mmHg to more than 10 times this value. These changes are less well documented in the deep posterior compartment, and here the pathological cause of the pain is not understood. The compartment syndrome affects the function of the knee indirectly because of its influence upon the use of the leg generally and the local pain experienced within the calf.

Although rest, alteration in training patterns and attention to shoe wear may prevent the symptoms of both 'shin splints' (or medial tibial syndrome) and compartment syndrome, certain cases will only respond to surgical decompression by means of a fasciotomy. This is very effective in the anterior compartment syndrome, but the results of surgery for 'shin splints' are less predictable.

Radionuclide scanning is usually negative, ruling out the presence of a tibial stress fracture. However, the deep compartment syndrome may be caused by a periostitis or chronic inflammatory condition along the medial tibial border where muscle attaches to bone, and in these cases the bone scan may be positive. Surgical release of this tissue can be effective in relieving some or all of the pain, but may have no effect upon muscle compartment pressure. On the other hand, the reduction in tissue pressure after fasciotomy of the anterior tibial compartment has been well documented.

Acute, post-traumatic compartment syndrome

Following fractures of the tibia, an acute compartment syndrome may affect the muscles of the calf, particularly if the fascia remains intact and there is no compounding of the fracture site. Soft-tissue pressure can be measured after tibial fractures and may increase to approximately 100 mmHg. If this is present for more than a few hours the function of muscle and nerve within the affected compartment will be seriously and permanently impaired.

The pathophysiology of the acute compartment syndrome involves a combination of:

- Arterial occlusion secondary to an increase in extravascular pressure brought about by haemorrhage
- Subsequent venous occlusion and stasis
- A superimposed soft-tissue oedema

The last process is produced in part by the release of vasocative amines, and these will compound the problems of the circulatory stasis by producing dilatation and increased capillary permeability. Muscle wet weight increases by over 50% and pressure receptors within the muscle fibres may in turn cause further arterial spasm.

The compartment syndrome is aggravated by systemic hypotension, increased metabolic rate and elevation of the affected limb. If relief of the acute syndrome is not ensured within 6 hours, and unremitting deep pain is the most significant presenting symptom, then the patient will be left with partial or complete paralysis of the affected muscles, patchy sensory loss and subsequent contractures affecting the foot. The presence or absence of a pulse cannot be used as a diagnostic feature, but pain on passive movement of the toes, distal pallor and cooling of the limb are significant additional features.

DEEP VENOUS THROMBOSIS

Clotting or thrombosis within the deep and superficial veins of the calf is caused by a combination of stasis of blood and injury to the vessel wall.

Lower limb fractures and other forms of significant trauma increase the likelihood of deep venous thrombosis. In addition, at least 50% of patients after lower limb surgery may also suffer from venous thrombosis. Calf swelling and chronic pain are the initial features, and the girths of the legs should be carefully compared. Oedema of the ankle and foot may develop and function of the knee and ankle are impaired.

If the thrombosis spreads proximally to involve the iliofemoral segment, there is an increased risk of a propagated clot, with subsequent pulmonary embolism. Lower limb injuries of any sort can produce thrombosis as far proximally as the pelvic veins, and the very real danger of a pulmonary embolism must be anticipated. Clinical detection of venous thrombosis is made possible by the use of venography, radioactive fibrinogen counting or Doppler ultrasound. However, many cases of deep vein thrombosis either go unnoticed or are missed, despite clinical examination.

If there is significant symptomatology and swelling of the leg, then anticoagulation is advisable with intravenous heparin initially for at least 48 hours until the concurrent use of oral warfarin affects the prothrombin time. In the older patient some degree of anticoagulation can be obtained with aspirin or dextran, although their prophylactic action is not marked.

PRESSURE SORES

These may be produced by tight plasters around the knee and lower portions of the leg. Local ischaemia produces microscopic changes within the skin and underlying tissues within 30 minutes, and shearing stress will extend the necrosis. At first the skin becomes erythematous. After 2 hours the changes become irreversible and the skin will then blister and become increasingly indurated.

The pressure sore extends deeply down to the underlying bone, such that a tetrahedron of necrotic fat underlies the affected skin. The necrosis may progress no further than to form a sterile abscess, but if infection then occurs an osteitis of bone may also develop. The skin ulcerates and its edges gradually become undermined such that major surgery may be necessary.

The simplest remedy for bed sores is to prevent their development. Tight plasters must be avoided and the regular turning of comatose or immobilized patients is an essential part of nursing and medical care of the injured.

References

Ahlbäck, S., Bauer, G.C.H. and Bohne, W.H. (1968) Spontaneous osteonecrosis of the knee. *Arthritis Rheum.*, **11**, 705–733

Aichroth, P.M. (1971) Osteochondritis dissecans of the knee. *J. Bone Joint Surg.*, **53B**, 440–447

Blount, W.P. (1937) Tibia vara : osteochondrosis deformans tibiae. *J. Bone Joint Surg.*, **19A**, 1–29

Bradley, J. and Dandy, D.J. (1989) Osteochondritis dissecans and other lesions of the femoral condyles. *J. Bone Joint Surg.*, **71B**, 518–522

Caffey, J., Madel, S.H., Roger, C. *et al* . (1958) Ossification of the distal femoral epiphysis. *J. Bone Joint Surg.*, **40A**, 467–474

Carey, R.P.L. (1983) Synovial chondromatosis of the knee in childhood. *J. Bone Joint Surg.*, **65B**, 444–447

Coolican, M.R. and Dandy, D.J. (1989) Arthroscopic management of synovial chondromatosis of the knee. Findings and results in 18 cases. *J. Bone Joint Surg.*, **71B**, 498–500

Daniel, D., Akeson, W., Amiel, D. *et al.* (1976) Lavage of septic joints in rabbits : effects of chondrolysis. *J. Bone Joint Surg.*, **58A**, 393–395

Edwards, D.H. and Bentley, G. (1977) Osteochondritis dissecans patellae. *J. Bone Joint Surg.*, **59B**, 58–63

Garrett, J.C. (1991) Osteochondritis dissecans. *Clin. Sports Med.*, **10**, 569–593

Gerhardt, M.C., Ready, J.E. and Mankin, H.J. (1990) Tumours about the knee in children. *Clin. Orthop.*, **225**, 86–110

Giron, V., Ganel, A. and Heim, M. (1991) Pigmented villonodular synovitis. *Arch. Dis. Childh.*, **66**, 1449–1450

Goldenberg, D.L., Brandt, K.D., Cohen, A.S. and Cathcart, E.S. (1975) Treatment of septic arthritis : comparison of needle aspiration and surgery as initial modes of joint drainage. *Arthritis Rheum.*, **18**, 83–90

Greene, W.B. (1993) Infantile tibia vara. *J. Bone Joint Surg.*, **73A**, 130–143

Hughston, J.C., Hergenroeder, P.T. and Courtenay, B.G. (1984) Osteochondritis dissecans of the femoral condyles. *J. Bone Joint Surg.*, **6A**, 1340–1348

Ivey, M. and Clark, R. (1985) Arthroscopic debridement of the knee for septic arthritis. *Clin. Orthop.*, **199**, 201–206

Jacobs, M.A., Loeb, P.E. and Hungerford, D.S. (1989) Core decompression of the distal femur for avascular necrosis of the knee. *J. Bone Joint Surg.*, **71B**, 583–587

Jarrett, M.P., Grossman, L., Sadler, A.H. and Grayzel, A.I. (1981) The role of arthroscopy in the treatment of septic arthritis. *Arthritis Rheum.*, **24**, 737–739

Joyce, M.J. and Mankin, H.J. (1983) Caveat arthroscopos : extra-articular lesions of bone simulating intra-articular pathology of the knee. *J. Bone Joint Surg.*, **65A**, 289–292

Juhl, M. and Krebs, B. (1989) Arthroscopy and synovial haemangioma or giant cell tumour of the knee. *Arch. Orthop. Trauma Surg.*, **108**, 250–252

Kistler, W. (1991) Synovial chondromatosis of the knee joint : a rarity during childhood. *Eur. J. Pediatr. Surg.*, **1**, 237–239

Klein, K.S., Aland, C.M., Kim, H.C. *et al.* (1987) Long-term follow-up of arthroscopic synovectomy for chronic hemophilic synovitis. *Arthroscopy*, **3**, 231–236

Koshino, T. (1982) The treatment of spontaneous osteonecrosis of the knee by high tibial osteotomy with and without bone-grafting or drilling of the lesion. *J. Bone Joint Surg.*, **64A**, 47–58

Koshino, T. and Okamoto, R. (1985) Resection of painful shelf (plica synovialis mediopatellaris) under arthroscopy. *Arthroscopy*, **1**, 136–141

Langenskiöld, A. (1981) Tibia vara : osteochondrosis deformans tibiae. *Clin. Orthop.*, **158**, 77–82

Limbird, T.J. and Dennis, S.C. (1987) Synovectomy and continuous passive motion (CPM) in hemophiliac patients. *Arthroscopy*, **3**, 74–79

Lindholm, S. and Pylkkänen, P. (1974) Internal fixation of the fragment of osteochondritis dissecans in the knee by means of bone pins : a preliminary report on several cases. *Acta Chir. Scand.*, **140**, 626–629

Lodwick, S., Wilson, A.J., Farrell, C. *et al.* (1980) Determining growth rates of focal bone lesions from radiographs. *Radiology*, **134**, 577–583

Macnicol, M.F. (1986) Osseous infection and immunodeficiency. In *Musculoskeletal*

Infections (eds Hughes, S.P.F. and Fitzgerald, R.H.), Year Book, Chicago, pp. 68–79

Motohashi, M., Morii, T. and Koshino, T. (1991) Clinical course and roentgeno-graphic changes of osteonecrosis in the femoral condyle under conservative treatment. *Clin. Orthop.*, **266**, 156–161

Ohl, M.D., Kean, J.R. and Steensen, R.N. (1991) Arthroscopic treatment of septic arthritic knees in children and adolescents. *Orthop. Rev.*, **20**, 894–896

Paget, J. (1870) On the production of some of the loose bodies in joints. *St. Bartholomew's Hospital Reports*, **6**, 1–4

Paley, D. and Jackson, R.W. (1986) Synovial haemangioma of the knee joint : diagnosis by arthroscopy. *Arthroscopy*, **2**, 174–177

Patel, D. (1986) Plica as a cause of anterior knee pain. *Orthop. Clin. North Am.*, **17**, 273–278

Petterson, H., Ahlberg, A. and Nilsson, I.M. (1980) A radiological classification of haemophilic arthropathy. *Clin. Orthop.*, **149**, 153–159

Pfeiffer, W.H., Gross, M.L. and Seeger, L.L. (1991) Osteochondritis dissecans of the patella. *Clin. Orthop.*, **271**, 207–211

Schoen, R.T., Aversa, J.M., Rahn, D.W. and Steere, A.C. (1991) Treatment of refractory chronic Lyme arthritis with arthroscopic synovectomy. *Arthritis Rheum.*, **34**, 1056–1060

Siffert, R.S. (1982) Intraepiphysial osteotomy for progressive tibia vara : case report and rationale of management. *J. Pediatr. Orthop.*, **2**, 81–85

Skyhar, M.J. and Mubarak, S.J. (1987) Arthroscopic treatment of septic knees in children. *J. Pediatr. Orthop.*, **7**, 647–651

Smillie, I.S. (1957) Treatment of osteochondritis dissecans. *J. Bone Joint Surg.*, **39B**, 248–260

Smith, J.B. (1990) Osteochondritis dissecans of the trochlea of the femur. *Arthroscopy*, **6**, 11–17

Stanitski, C.L., Harvell, J.C. and Fu, F.H. (1989) Arthroscopy in acute septic knees. Management in pediatric patients. *Clin. Orthop.*, **241**, 209–212

Thomson, N.L. (1987) Osteochondritis dissecans and osteochondral fragments managed by Herbert compression screw fixation. *Clin. Orthop.*, **224**, 71–78

Twyman, R.S., Desai, K. and Aichroth, P.M. (1991) Osteochondritis dissecans of the knee : a long-term study. *J. Bone Joint Surg.*, **73B**, 461–464

Weidel, J.D. (1990) Arthroscopy of the knee in hemophilia. *Prog. Clin. Biol. Res.*, **324**, 231–239

Wilson, J.N. (1967) A diagnostic sign in osteochondritis of the knee. *J. Bone Joint Surg.*, **49A**, 477–480

10
Treatment of soft-tissue injuries

STAGES OF HEALING – TYPE I FIBRE – TYPE II FIBRE –
THERAPY – KNEE BRACING – ULTRASOUND –
INTERFERENTIAL THERAPY – MASSAGE AND
MANIPULATION – HEAT – ANALGESIC THERAPY –
PATHOLOGICAL CONDITIONS AFFECTING MUSCLE –
CONCLUSION

ACUTE INJURY

Acute soft tissue injuries occur from direct (extrinsic) or indirect (intrinsic) trauma. Collision with another player, the ground or a fixed object will produce typical patterns of damage, although the precise extent of the injury may be difficult to ascertain. Indirect injuries from forced rotation and rapid stretch or deceleration may be harder to diagnose, although the site of discomfort is usually localized. A third category of injury is the 'overuse syndrome' where repetitive submaximal stresses exceed the resilience of structures comprising the joint.

Whenever ligament, tendon, muscle or bone are injured acutely, blood vessels are disrupted at the site of the tear or fracture. The resultant haemorrhage within the confined space produces a haematoma, from which spring the cells of regeneration or repair. Whether the deficiency is made good by scar or by a restitution of the normal tissue, the cellular response progresses through the stages of inflammation, proliferation, remodelling and maturation. Excessive early movement and inappropriate loading may retard this process, as will the presence of gapping, inadequate nutrition and oxygenation, and infection.

Inflammation

The central and peripheral mediators of inflammation interact in a complex fashion, their concentrations being controlled by the activation of precursors, often through cascade reactions, and the subsequent recruitment of inhibitors and inactivating enzymes. The vasodilatatory response is mediated by histamine, bradykinin, prostaglandin and other evanescent substances such as 5-hydroxytryptamine. Blood clot acts as an early scaffold, filling the gap in a ligament tear with coagulum which gradually builds up collagen type III, and later collagen type I as the long-term matrix (Woo and Buckwalter, 1987). Chronic inflammatory tissue subsequently aggregates glycosaminoglycan, fibronectin and DNA, and these in turn delineate the early formation of the host tissue.

Proliferation

Differentiation of the cellular morphology progresses in parallel with the establishment of a definitive blood supply. Although water content remains elevated compared to normal tissue, there is a progressive change in the constituents of the tissue, including increased concentrations of type I collagen and extracellular matrix. The architecture of the healing tissue remains immature, as in callus formation at a fracture, but a gradual reorientation of the constituent fibres occurs, particularly if subjected to controlled loading.

Remodelling and maturation

Over several months the collagen turnover rate returns to normal and the macroscopic shape of the healing tissue becomes better defined. The extracellular matrix is restored, although it may never return entirely to normal (Figure 10.1). A mature and efficient blood supply is established, allowing the return of gliding movement to ligament and tendon if scarring is broken down progressively. However, the return of a competent nerve supply of afferent neurons is rarely achieved in full (Johansson *et al.*, 1991), so that the repaired tissue may remain chronically susceptible to re-injury. This should be remembered when advising the patient about a return to sport after ligament reconstruction and emphasizes the importance of training other components of normal lower limb function.

Wasting of the type I muscle fibres, the so-called 'slow' fibres which are responsible for muscle tone, results from disuse and characterizes injuries to the knee where there is loss of joint movement or a lack of exercise owing to pain. Rupture of ligaments such as the anterior cruciate will also reduce the proprioceptive input (Barrett, 1991; Corrigan *et al.*, 1992) and the stimulus for muscle development. Occasionally, a primary abnormality of muscle is present, such as a myopathy or myositis ossificans, and wasting is also associated with conditions such as rheumatoid arthritis, haemophilic arthropathy and certain neurological disorders.

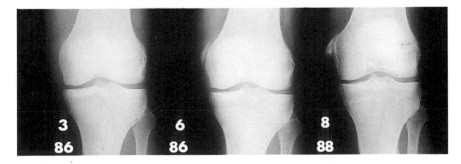

Figure 10.1 *Ossification developing after a tear of the femoral attachment of the medial collateral ligament*

Type I muscle fibre

The type I or slow-twitch fibre is low in adenosine triphosphatase (ATP-ase) and glycolytic enzymes, and is dependent upon aerobic metabolism. This reliance upon oxidative metabolism is demonstrated histologically by an increase in mitochondrial enzymes, and the large number of capillaries which supply this muscle type. Although type I fibres are more resistant to fatigue, they atrophy rapidly if the knee is immobilized and are not well preserved by isometric contractions. The population of type I fibres within a muscle seems to be genetically determined and is probably little influenced by physical training.

Type II muscle fibre

The type II or fast-twitch fibre is characterized by a high ATP-ase content and a greater degree of glycolytic enzymic activity than is seen in the type I fibre. Type II fibres have been subdivided into groups A, B, C and M

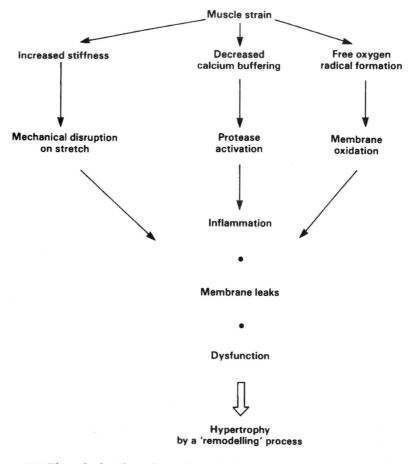

Figure 10.2 *The pathophysiology of a muscle strain. Muscle strain and microtears usually result from the rapid lengthening of activated muscles (eccentric contraction). Injury is proportional to the maximum tension generated and the extent of muscle fatigue*

(Gauthier, 1986). The fast-twitch type IIA (fast/red myosin) fibres possess some oxidative capacity owing to the presence of mitochondria and myoglobin and are therefore more resistant to fatigue than the type IIB (fast/white myosin) fibres which are completely glycolytic (anaerobic). Type IIC are intermediate fibres comprising a mixture of types A and B, while a recently identified Type IIM ('superfast') fibre contains a specific myosin.

Training by means of specific muscle exercises will produce variable improvement in strength and endurance. High-tension, low-frequency contractions stimulate hypertrophy, particularly of the type II fibres (Faulkner, 1986), and the stimulus of stretch is also beneficial. Eccentric contraction (activation of the muscle while it is being lengthened by an opposing force greater than the force in the muscle) replicates the demand placed upon muscle very effectively and is recognized to be a vital component of rehabilitation or training. The tension developed in eccentrically loaded muscle is greater than during isometric loading, and considerably greater than in concentric contraction. Hence muscle is frequently injured during peaks of eccentric contraction (Figure 10.2), usually failing in the region of the myotendinous junction. Conversely, metabolic efficiency is greatest with concentric and least with eccentric contraction.

Low-tension, repetitive exercise improves endurance, but when training is discontinued the number of oxidative fibres regresses to the control value within weeks. Although isometric exercises may prevent the atrophy of type II fibres, particularly the type II B group, endurance training has no effect upon cross-sectional size of muscle. Instead, it increases the number of capillaries per muscle fibre, and possibly the levels of oxidative enzymes. Conversely, resistive training using weights increases the size of muscle fibres and thereby their strength, but there is no increase in their oxidative capacity.

THERAPY

The rule of 12s

In the first *12 seconds* after injury the decision is made to stop a player from participating further. The assessment must be hurried but informed, and may involve the team coach, physiotherapist or doctor. Pain, laxity and deformity are judged as accurately as possible. Inability to weightbear and loss of movement are absolute contraindications to continuing with the sport.

During the next *12 minutes* the player is reassessed off the field. Generally the decision to stop playing is consolidated and severe injuries should be protected with a temporary splint. Haemorrhage, whether revealed or concealed, is controlled with compression and cooling.

Over the ensuing *12 hours* rest, ice, compression and elevation are time-honoured remedies. Fractures should be ruled out by radiographs and the player referred to a surgeon if skeletal or soft tissue injuries merit this.

Cooling by ice packs, a frozen pea packet, a silicone gel bag or cold water compress limits the inflammatory response, principally by constricting the capillaries supplying the injured tissue. The applications should be for approximately 20 minutes every 2 hours and a Cryocuff (Aircast Incorp., Summit, N.J.) will also ensure gentle compression. Alternatively, pressure may be applied evenly over the knee by Tubigrip or bandaging. Rest and elevation are ensured by instructing the athlete to keep the leg with 'toes above your nose', since this makes up for the lack of muscle pump in the resting limb. Splintage with a backshell canvas support or light brace will relieve pain when abnormal laxity is present, and anti-inflammatory analgesics are prescribed.

The first *12 days* after the injury are spent controlling the inflammation further and preserving the range of movement without incurring additional damage. With haematoma and swelling limited, the joint should be reassessed. Many injuries occur on a Saturday and therefore this examination is carried out on a Sunday or a Monday. Pain is inhibitory and Hilton's law of rest and pain (Hilton, 1863) is still valid, requiring the patient to remain at rest at least over the weekend. The therapist gains further insight into the severity of the injury over these 12 days, and referral for a surgical opinion is best achieved during this time.

The *12-week* phase concentrates on regaining mobility, power and normal function. The speed of recovery will vary according to the injury (Durand *et al.*, 1993) and the rapport established between the patient and physiotherapist. Important characteristics of the patient are motivation, expectations, general fitness and physique. Hypermobility or lack of flexibility should be noted, together with alignment of the leg and foot posture. Training and return to sport is usually achieved even if surgical intervention has been necessary.

Following severe injuries, particularly cruciate ligament disruption and displaced fractures, a *12-month* rehabilitation period is usual before sport can be continued. Loss of agility, co-ordination and confidence takes time to recover, even if the range of movement and muscle bulk have been restored more rapidly. The complex interplay between psyche and motor skills will be understood by the experienced coach and therapist. Communication, reassurance and altered training patterns help towards full rehabilitation.

In summary, the aims of therapy are:

- to preserve strength without undue stress to the injured part
- to maintain or restore the normal range of motion
- to preserve patellar mobility
- to regain proprioception and agility
- to recover endurance or confidence
- to return to full functional activity

Specific elements in physiotherapy have become better defined in the last few years, particularly the postoperative regimen following anterior cruciate ligament reconstruction (Figures 10.3 and 10.4a,b). Based on the premise that a relatively rapid return of full movement and normal gait is beneficial, this 'accelerated rehabilitation' (Shelbourne and Nitz, 1990) was conceived in response to the observation that 'non-compliant' patients made a more rapid and complete recovery than those who followed the suggested protocol of a guarded and delayed return of movement and power. It was also noted that complications such as stiffness and anterior

1 As swelling decreases, movement should increase

2 Weightbearing and 'closed kinetic chain' exercises return the limb to normal use
   (a) 0–4 weeks – partial weightbearing with 10–90° flexion arc
   (b) 4–16 weeks – increase to full weightbearing and 0–135° of flexion

3 Normal gait should be achieved by 4–6 weeks

4 The appearance of the scar offers a monitor of the degree of graft maturation

5 The KT-1000 arthrometer (see Figure 10.4a,b) allows the assessment of residual laxity
   at 6–18 months postoperatively (65 mm or less compared to the normal knee)

6 A graduated return to sport is permitted over 6–18 months postoperatively in the expec-
   tation that 90% of patients will achieve this

Figure 10.3 *Monitoring progress after anterior cruciate ligament reconstruction*

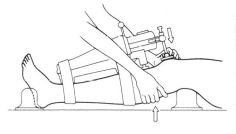

(a)

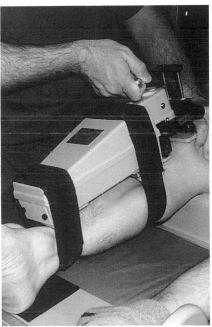

Figure 10.4(a,b) *The KT-1000 arthrometer*   (b)

knee pain were uncommon in those who recovered rapidly. However, it is equally possible that those who progressed quickly were a self-selected group where motivation, problem-free surgery and muscle recovery combined to produce a good result. Until a prospective trial reveals the long-term results to be convincingly better, accelerated physiotherapy cannot be supported unconditionally.

Pain

The relief of pain in the immediate postoperative period can be achieved by epidural or regional anaesthesia, opiate analgesia and by continuous passive motion (CPM) (Noyes *et al.*, 1987; Paulos *et al.*, 1991). If a CPM machine is used when there is potential anterolateral laxity, anterior translation of the proximal tibia should be minimized by avoiding the use of a support behind the upper calf (Drez *et al.*, 1991). Transcutaneous electrical nerve stimulation (TENS) and cooling the joint with a Cryocuff (Aircast) will also give temporary pain relief.

Strength

Agonist-antagonist control   Muscle strength is maintained by active-assistance range of movement initially, which may be all that a painful lesion will permit. Co-contraction of the extensor and flexor muscle groups is encouraged as a means of stabilizing the joint where pathological laxity is present, or as a means of protecting a graft reconstruction of a ligament. Each therapist will develop an individualistic approach to the stages of rehabilitation, but it is now widely recognized that supervised movement should be allowed immediately. Strength is later developed by bringing in eccentric as well as concentric muscle contraction.

Quadriceps 'setting' can be achieved with both isometric and isotonic exercises, and in the early stages taping or strapping (Figure 10.5a–c) will lessen pain by improving patellar tracking (McConnell, 1986) or knee stability. 'Inner range' quadriceps drill, emphasizing vastus medialis power, is achieved by combining knee extension with adduction of the externally rotated leg; retropatellar pain is often controlled by confining the early stages of therapy to isometric contraction of vastus medialis with the knee flexed at varying angles and the thigh rotated externally. A graduated approach to regaining power is particularly important in patellar pain syndromes where confidence must be restored if lasting relief of pain is to be achieved.

Eccentric contraction stimulates muscle hypertrophy, essential in sports requiring sudden deceleration such as jumping, downhill 'fell' running and cycling. Plyometrics encourages eccentric power and control, but may not be appropriate for bulky athletes engaged in power sports. This decision lies with the physiotherapist and emphasizes the importance of tailoring exercises to the physique and sporting demands of the patient.

Electrically induced co-contraction of the thigh muscles (Wigerstand-Lossing *et al.*, 1988; Snyder-Mackler *et al.*, 1991) has yet to find a significant role in rehabilitation, and as a general principle conscious effort by the patient is preferable. Nevertheless, if an impasse is reached in the early stages of an exercise programme, both electrical stimulation and CPM may have a limited role to play. Manipulation under anaesthesia may also regain motion in the later stages of recovery if stiffness and a block to extension or flexion become established.

Closed kinetic chain exercises   The changing concepts in rehabilitation after anterior cruciate reconstruction have been described by Reid (1993). There has been a move away from unloaded, knee extension work. These 'open kinetic chain' exercises were conducted with the foot in a free (non-stationary) position and placed considerable anterior tibial translational and

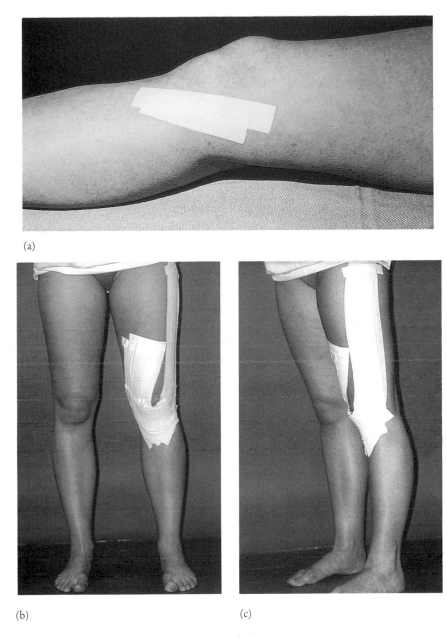

(a)

(b)   (c)

Figure 10.5 Supportive taping (a) or strapping (b,c)

patellofemoral forces through the knee (Grood *et al.*, 1984). Closed kinetic chain exercises, with the foot fixed, are therefore preferred as they promote maximal joint stability and co-contraction of the quadriceps and hamstring groups (Palmitier *et al.*, 1991). It is also preferable to increase the time spent on these exercises rather than emphasizing progressive loading. Leg presses are preferred to standard knee extension drill against resistance (Grood *et al.*, 1984) and the dangers of single episodes of excessive loading or cyclical shearing stress guarded against (Reid, 1993).

Closed chain exercises are a more natural means of training and markedly improve endurance. Stair climbing, stationary bicycling, the rowing machine and jogging offer individual patients a welcome relief from repeated single exercises and encourage a sense of improvement. Step-ups, both forwards and sideways, with eyes open and then closed, provide a simple means of monitoring the return of precision activity (Macnicol, 1992) and agility can be improved with the use of a wobble board or small trampoline. Initially the patient concentrates on simple balance, but later in the programme a second activity, such as catching and throwing a ball, is introduced, while the patient stands on the injured leg.

Compression bandaging is permissible if this gives confidence and a greater sense of knee control. When discomfort and insecurity are marked, exercises in a warm swimming pool are confidence-boosting and reduce loading and torque stress through the knee. General fitness should be developed, especially power in the opposite leg, upper body strength and cardiorespiratory reserve.

Flexibility

Alongside muscle strengthening should be a programme of stretching tight structures such as the iliotibial band, the hamstrings and the calf. Tensor fasciae latae (Figure 10.6) is often adaptively shortened, and distal contracture of the iliotibial band is reversed by medial patellar translocation with the patient in a side-lying position. Stretching exercises should also be taught routinely as part of a 'warm-up' and a 'warm-down'. Once again, closed chain exercises and a progressive return to weightbearing are now recognized as important components of restoring flexibility, taken in conjunction with the minimal use of external splint or brace support.

Warm-up is known to reduce muscle viscosity, manifest by both improved contraction and greater elasticity. Stretching should be conducted after a warm-up, slowly and regularly over time. This will gradually ease muscle tightness and will enhance conditioning. Musculotendinous tears are more common in the two joint units (hamstrings, rectus femoris and gastrocnemius), so particular attention should be paid to their stretching, both after warm up and during cool-down. In this way soft-tissue injuries should be minimized (Ekstrand and Gillquist, 1982; Garrett *et al.*, 1984).

Gait

Re-education will involve a change in gait pattern which has developed in response to a chronic instability. Adaptation following ligament injury was investigated by Perry *et al.* (1980) when they reviewed the intended effects of pes anserinus transfer, using gait analysis and electromyography. Stride length, single limb support time and walking speed were uniformly reduced, and the effects of pesplasty were not considered to be significantly therapeutic.

A 'quadriceps–avoidance' gait was observed by Berchuck *et al.* (1991) in patients with an absent anterior cruciate ligament. The magnitude of flexion was appreciably reduced during walking or jogging, thus preventing anterior translation of the proximal tibia by the relatively unopposed effect

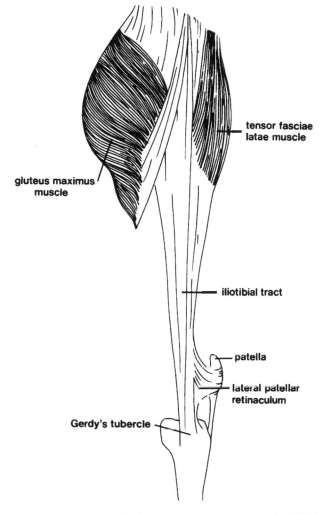

Figure 10.6 *Tensor fasciae latae (and gluteus maximus) inserts into the tibia but also into the patella and the lateral femoral condyle*

of quadriceps contraction. Climbing stairs was unaffected by this alteration and 25% of their patients did not adopt a quadriceps-avoidance gait. The combination of anterior cruciate deficiency and varus alignment leads to an abnormally high moment of adduction with medial shift of loading through the joint (Noyes *et al.*, 1992). Quadriceps inhibition was also noted, with a reduction of extensor muscle force and enhanced hamstring muscle activity in approximately half of the group under study. Degenerative changes are more likely, therefore, when laxity is combined with varus deformity.

Isokinetics

Over the past 25 years isokinetic devices have been developed into complex machines such as the Biodex, Cybex and KinCom. The principle behind isokinetic exercise is that an accommodating resistance should be applied to

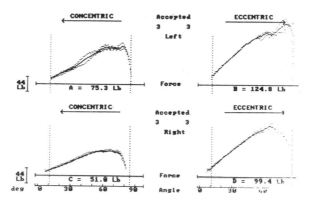

Figure 10.7 A KinCom read-out, comparing the quadriceps power of the normal left leg and the injured right leg

a limb moving at a fixed speed or angular velocity. Maximal or submaximal load can therefore be ensured at all angles in the range of movement.

Muscle function can be quantified by providing data on peak torque, average torque, work expended and power developed. Muscle contraction can be divided into the concentric and eccentric phases (Figure 10.7) with a high degree of retest reliability. The objective measurements allow comparison between the normal and abnormal limb after injury, and offer the physiotherapist both the means of monitoring recovery and of providing a structured and progressive programme of resisted exercises. Hence the patient can be closely supervised after injury or reconstruction of the anterior cruciate ligament, as a common example, and an optimum ratio between quadriceps and hamstring power is established. Hamstring strength of some 70% of quadriceps strength may be increased by hamstring drill if anterolateral knee laxity requires greater dynamic control. Accessories for each machine also allow closed kinetic chain exercises as a means of enhancing rehabilitation. The aim is to restore power in the injured leg to within 10% of the normal side.

KNEE BRACING

The value of knee bracing is unproven, and their use prophylactically, as has been suggested for children in certain sports, is unwarranted (Grace *et al.*, 1988). Much depends upon the compliance of the patient and the brace may offer little more than an improvement in proprioception (Cook *et al.*, 1989). Stark (1850) is reported to have made the first knee brace, describing, in an Edinburgh journal, the use of a steel spring for two patients.

The problems inherent in bracing include:

- Awkward design and bulk
- Unacceptable weight
- Restrictive of flexion and rapid movement
- Friction over points of contact

- Compression and the production of localized oedema
- Translation

Migration of the orthosis remains a significant problem and can only be minimized by custom-made braces. Beck *et al.* (1986) studied seven brands of functional knee braces and found that anterior tibial translation could not be prevented when peak forces were applied to a level typical of strenuous sport. Control of rotational forces is enhanced, but this effect is greater at 60° than at 30° of flexion (Wojtys *et al.*, 1987), and therefore the derotational effect on the extended, weightbearing joint is probably minimal.

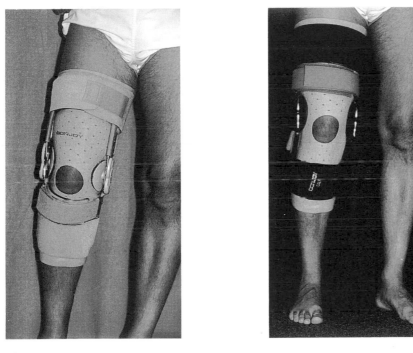

(a)

Figure 10.8 A Don Joy brace designed to support the knee after anterior cruciate ligament reconstruction (a) and to control posterior cruciate chronic laxity (b)

The new generation of braces (Figure 10.8a,b) impedes activity less, in contrast to earlier concerns about the constraints upon normal knee motion (Houston and Gœmans, 1982). Approximately one-half of anterior cruciate-deficient knees are improved by bracing, judged by the protection against episodes of giving way, swelling and pain. Combined ligament injuries may also be supported effectively in the early stages of recuperation. Cawley *et al.* (1991) reviewed a large number of papers dealing with the use of braces, noting that at least 25 commercial braces are available. Objective assessment and scientifically convincing data were rare, but the overall impression gained was that bracing is of value both as a means of improving proprioception and by the stabilizing effect (Figure 10.9).

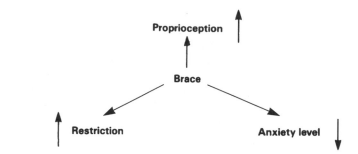

Figure 10.9 The therapeutic effects of bracing

ULTRASOUND

Ultrasound produces a local increase in tissue temperature and may alter the biochemical structure of collagen. This improves flexibility and the treatment is therefore valuable in the later stages of management of soft-tissue trauma, such as sprains and strains, tendonitis, bursitis, and joint stiffness. A combination of ultrasound and electrical muscle stimulation may speed recovery after a limb has been immobilized, but muscle re-education still depends largely upon voluntary effort.

INTERFERENTIAL THERAPY

Deeper, and more directed, electrical therapy can be provided by the 'cross-fire' effect of two currents directed at right angles to each other. This is thought to inhibit the parasympathetic system if high frequencies, over 4000 Hertz, are used. At lower frequencies the muscle may be stimulated to contract, and this is not necessarily of value. Both interferential therapy and ultrasound have a part to play, but must not be used by unskilled attendants.

MASSAGE AND MANIPULATION

The use of massage is controversial and it may often be abused. Frictional massage, where the fingertips apply firm pressure across the line of a muscle or tendon, may break down adhesions and can be combined with stretching exercises. Vibratory massage may also be beneficial, if only to relieve symptoms; but deep and firm massage can be injurious to inflamed or recovering muscles. In the early stages of the rehabilitation after injury, therefore, massage must be used with care.

Manipulation of a stiffened knee joint is sometimes justified and may restore a better range of movement. However, the causes of restricted movement should be ruled out and excessive manipulation may damage a meniscus or other structure within the knee. Complete relaxation of the patient is necessary and therefore a general anaesthetic is occasionally indicated. The technique is not recommended in the athlete and great care must be taken to avoid further injury.

HEAT

Heat in the form of short-wave diathermy, which allows a deeper permeation of the rays, is occasionally recommended when a muscle is recovering from injury. However, radiant heat (hot water bottles, heat lamps or liniments) or short-wave diathermy are not recommended in the early stages after an injury as they may increase the hyperaemic response. It is far better to rely upon rest and cooling for the tissues initially.

When scar tissue has formed, there may be a place for increasing tissue temperature and thus improving blood flow and the possibility of scar breakdown. Heat also has a sedative and analgesic effect which may allow greater muscle stretching and reduce spasm.

ANALGESIC THERAPY

Apart from the use of anti-inflammatory analgesics (Figure 10.10), transcutaneous electrical stimulation can also reduce the perception of pain. The small nerve fibres conducting pain impulses are thought to be blocked at

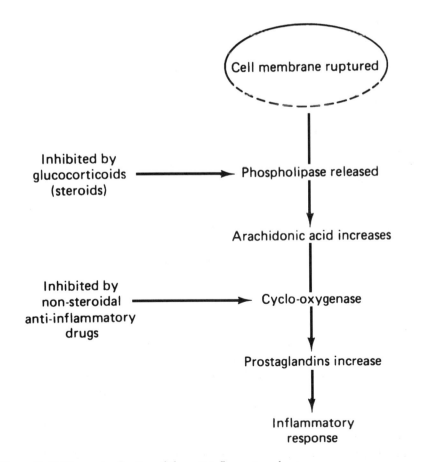

Figure 10.10 The mode of action of the anti-inflammatory drugs

the level of the spinal cord and there may be an increased release of pain-inhibiting substances, such as endorphins and encephalins.

The lessening in pain experienced by the patient after injury will permit an earlier return to exercise and joint movement, but there is always the risk that further damage may be incurred. The same criticism can be levelled at the use of ice or various other forms of cryotherapy, including ethylchloride 'cold' spray, which may deaden the sensitivity of nerves but at the same time make the knee more vulnerable to further injury.

PATHOLOGICAL CONDITIONS AFFECTING MUSCLE

Partial tear or complete rupture of muscle

Partial tear or complete rupture of the belly or musculotendinous region of a muscle is not uncommon and may affect the quadriceps, hamstring, adductor or calf muscle groups. The formation of an interstitial haematoma, or an intramuscular bleed, will obviously restrict the function of that muscle and produce pain. Indirectly, the knee is thus involved. Rarely, muscle may also be avulsed from its point of attachment in bone, and occasionally it should therefore be reattached. Generally, however, suturing a muscle rupture is unwise and will not benefit the patient.

Treatment should be directed at reducing the formation of scar by rest and local cooling. Later, when the scar has become mature, it can be gently stretched and muscle function returned to a near-normal level.

Contracture of muscle

Contracture occurs when the muscle is allowed to shorten, and hence works from a reduced resting length. Contracture is common after disuse or inflammatory conditions involving joints, and will also occur if there is a muscle imbalance, as is seen in certain neuromuscular abnormalities. With the passage of time, the contracture tends to worsen and although physiotherapy may partially correct the shortened length, a residual deficit is usually present.

Compartment syndrome

This may be either acute or chronic. In the former, trauma produces an increased pressure within the fascial compartment surrounding muscle, part of the haemorrhage very commonly occurring as a result of fracture. Tissue pressure increases as a result of arterial haemorrhage, venostasis and the resultant oedema. Intravascular pressure is rapidly exceeded and muscle and related segments of nerve become ischaemic.

In the chronic form, repetitive activity produces pressure, inflammation and possibly a metabolic acidosis in muscle, and this in turn results in swelling. If the muscle is not free to expand, pressure rises and will impair the blood supply to the muscle with increasing pain as metabolites build up within the muscle. Although symptoms are quickly relieved by rest, they may prove very limiting. An adhesive tendonitis may be difficult to differentiate from chronic muscle compartment syndrome.

Myositis ossificans

Myositis ossificans describes a pathological process whereby calcification tales place, leading eventually to mature bone formation within the damaged area of a rupture or partially torn muscle. Calcium deposits within the haematoma and the deposition of bone may be increased by a rapid resumption of activity. In particular, the stretching of muscle may stimulate the ossification process and lead to increasing disability.

Excision of 'mature' ossified deposits is occasionally advocated, but there is a tendency for the myositis ossificans to recur. Although the process may be affected by certain drugs, the principal treatment of the condition is the restriction of its occurrence by using a graduated and careful programme of convalescence.

Occasionally muscle may be infected by inadvised injections, or cysts and fibrocytic nodules may form within the thigh. The principal method of treatment is prevention, but if these do occur, medical attention is essential and a surgical drainage procedure may be required.

Muscular dystrophy

Muscular dystrophy may be a cause for muscle wasting, and various neurological and muscular conditions should always by considered in a patient whose recovery appears abnormal, or if wasting of groups of muscles become progressive.

Reflex sympathetic dystrophy

This condition has also been termed causalgia, alyodystrophy or Sudeck's atrophy. Injury or surgery are precipitants and it is characterised by a burning pain, often widespread around the knee, which persists at night. Numbness, stiffness, mechanical symptoms and swelling may occur in varying degrees to confuse the clinical picture (Tietjen, 1986). Skin changes include discolouration, sweating, change in temperature and sensory alteration. The vasomotor changes involve deeper tissues so that stiffness and radiographic rarefaction of bone occur (Seale, 1989).

Knee stiffness and weakness initially result from the pain produced during muscle action and joint movement, but eventually oedema and fibrosis lead to a more morbid process. The nociceptive nerve fibres contain substance P which can be mapped by immunohistochemistry (Wotjys *et al.*, 1990), while an inflammatory process is confirmed by increased uptake on radioisotope bone scanning, especially during the first six months of the condition. The anterior knee pain syndromes may also be associated with a positive scan and these sympathetically-mediated symptoms are best dealt with non-surgically. Thermography (Plate 47) in the vasodilatory, acute stage of the condition confirms an increase in temperature of 2–3°C and may be used to monitor the response to treatment (Rothschild, 1990).

Reflex sympathetic dystrophy is conventionally divided into an acute, early phase characterised by pain, then by a dystrophic phase where stiffness and sympathetic over-activity are obvious, and a final, often intractable stage. Stiffness may become established and is complicated by the secondary changes of muscle wasting and arthrofibrosis. In some patients a gradual improvement occurs with time, with a slow return to normal activity. In others, the joint becomes permanently restricted and painful, compounded by anxiety or depression.

Treatment of the dystrophy will be more successful if it is recognised early. In-patient physiotherapy, non-steroidal anti-inflammatory analgesia and sometimes counselling are important components in preventing the progression of the stages towards irreversible stiffness. Intervention and forcible manipulation are contra-indicated but arthroscopic irrigation and sympathetic blockade by pharmacological agents should be considered if an extensive exercise programme fails. Continuous epidural anaesthesia using an indwelling catheter for four days was described by Cooper *et al.* (1989) who were then able to establish continuous passive motion. This form of management relieves the symptoms in approximately two-thirds of patients although its timing may be critical. Regional intravenous guanethidine blocks are also effective (Bonelli *et al.*, 1983).

CONCLUSION

Throughout this book emphasis has been placed upon the importance of a practical approach to injuries of the knee, based upon anatomical knowledge and appreciation of the interrelationship between muscle, ligament and joint function. When a soft-tissue injury or fracture occurs there is a concomitant loss of movement and of muscle power during the stages of healing. Treatment should be directed towards a return of normal movement and muscle strength, but should not hasten events to the extent that an effusion recurs or ligament laxity is promoted. Obstructive lesions within the knee should be recognized early, by careful clinical examination and appropriate investigation, and removed before the articulating surfaces of the knee are damaged.

The experienced coach, physiotherapist or doctor will have learnt that recovery from injury also depends upon the general fitness and motivation of the athlete or patient. Success attends the two-way process where the patient respects the skills and recommendations of the therapist, and where the therapist in turn trusts to the efforts of his charge.

References

Barrett, D.S. (1991) Proprioception and function after anterior cruciate reconstruction. *J. Bone Joint Surg.*, **73B**, 833–837

Beck, C., Drez, D., Young, J. *et al.* (1986) Instrumental testing of functional knee braces. *Am. J. Sports Med.*, **14**, 253–255

Berchuck, M., Andriacchi, T.P. and Bach, B.R. (1991) Gait adaptations by patients who have a deficient anterior cruciate ligament. *J. Bone Joint Surg.*, **72A**, 871–877

Bonelli, S., Conoscente, F., Morilia, A. *et al.* (1983) Regional intravenous guanethidine vs stellate ganglion block in reflex sympathetic dystrophies: a randomised trial. *Pain*, **16**, 297–307

Cawley, P.W., France, P. and Paulos, L.E. (1991) The current state of functional knee bracing research. *Am. J. Sports Med.*, **19**, 226–233

Cook, F.F., Tibone, J.E. and Redfern, F.C. (1989) A dynamic analysis of a functional brace for anterior cruciate insufficiency. *Am. J. Sports Med.*, **17**, 519–524

Cooper, D.E., De Lec, J.C. and Ramamurthy, S. (1989) Reflex sympathetic dystrophy of the knee. Treatment using continuous epidural anaesthesia. *J. Bone Joint Surg.*, **71B**, 365–369

Corrigan, J.P., Cashman, W.F. and Brady, M.P. (1992) Proprioception in the cruciate deficient knee. *J. Bone Joint Surg.*, **74B**, 247–250

Drez, D., Paine, R.M., Neuschwander, D.C. and Young, J.C. (1991) *In vivo* measurement of anterior tibial translation using continuous passive motion devices. *Am. J. Sport Med.*, **19**, 381–383

Durand, A., Richards, C.L., Malouin, F. and Bravo, G. (1993) Motor recovery after arthroscopic partial meniscectomy. *J. Bone Joint Surg.*, **7A**, 202–214

Ekstrand, J. and Gillquist, J. (1982) The frequency of muscle tightness and injuries in soccer players. *Am. J. Sports Med.*, **10**, 75–78

Faulkner, J.A. (1986) New perspectives in training for maximum performance. *J. Am. Med. Ass.*, **205**, 741–746

Garrett, W.E. Jr, Califf, J.C. and Bassett, F.H. (1984) Histochemical correlates of hamstring injuries. *Am. J. Sports Med.*, **12**, 98–103

Gauthier, G.F. (1986) Skeletal muscle fiber types. In *Myology*, Vol. 1 (eds Engel, A.G. and Banker, B.Q.), McGraw-Hill, New York, pp. 255–284

Grace, T.G., Skipper, B.J., Newberry, J.C. et al. (1988) Prophylactic knee braces and injury to the lower extremity. *J. Bone Joint Surg.*, **70A**, 422–427

Grood, E.S., Suntag, J., Noyes, F.R. and Butler, D.l. (1984) Biomechanics of the knee extension exercise. Effect of cutting the anterior cruciate ligament. *J. Bone Joint Surg.*, **66A**, 725–734

Hilton, J. (1863) *The Influence of Mechanical and Physiological Rest*, Bell and Daldy, London

Houston, M.E. and Goemans, P.H. (1982) Leg muscle performance of athletes with and without knee support braces. *Arch. Phys. Med. Rehabil.*, **63**, 431–432

Johansson, H., Sjolander, P. and Sojka, P. (1991) A sensory role for the cruciate ligaments. *Clin. Orthop.*, **268**, 161–178

McConnell, J. (1986) The management of chondromalacia patellae. a long-term solution. *Aust. J Physiother.*, **32**, 215–224

Macnicol, M.F. (1992) The conservative management of the anterior cruciate ligament-deficient knee. In *Knee Surgery : Current Practice* (eds Aichroth, P.M. and Dilworth Cannon, W.), Martin Dunitz, London, pp. 217–221

Noyes, F.R., Mangine, R.E. and Barber, S. (1987) Early knee motion after open and arthroscopic anterior cruciate ligament reconstruction. *Am. J. Sports Med.*, **15**, 149–160

Noyes, F.R., Schipplein, O.D., Andriacchi, T.P. et al. (1992) The anterior cruciate ligament-deficient knee with varus alignment. An analysis of gait adaptations and dynamic joint loadings. *Am. J. Sports Med.*, **20**(6), 707–716

Palmitier, R.A., Kai-Nan, A., Scott, S.G. and Chao, E.Y.S. (1991) Kinetic chain exercise in knee rehabilitation. *Sports Med*, **II**, 404–413

Paulos, L.E., Wnorowski, D.C. and Beck, C.L. (1991) Rehabilitation following knee surgery. *Sports Med*, **II**, 257–275

Perry, J., Fox, J.M. and Boitano, M.A. (1980) Functional evaluation of the pes anserinus transfer by electromyography and gait analysis. *J. Bone Joint Surg.*, **62A**, 973–980

Reid, D.C. (1993) Current concepts in rehabilitation of the anterior cruciate deficient knee. *Curr. Orthopaedics*, **7**, 101–105

Rothschild, B. (1990) Reflex sympathetic dystrophy. *Arthritis Care Res.*, **3**, 144–153

Seale, K. (1989) Reflex sympathetic dystrophy of the lower extremity. *Clin. Orthop.*, **243**, 80–85

Shelbourne, K.D. and Nitz, P. (1990) Accelerated rehabilitation after anterior cruciate ligament reconstruction. *Am. J. Sports Med.*, **80**, 292–299

Snyder-Meckler, L., Ladin, Z., Shepsis, A.A. and Young, J.C. (1991) Electrical stimulation of the thigh muscles after reconstruction of the anterior cruciate ligament. *J. Bone Joint Surg.*, **73A**, 1025–1036

Stark, J. (1850) Two cases of rupture of the crucial ligaments of the knee joint. *Edinb. Med. Surg.*, **74**, 267–271

Tietjen, B. (1986) Reflex sympathetic dystrophy of the knee. *Clin. Orthop.*, **209**, 234–243

Wigerstad-Lossing, I., Grimby, G., Johsson, T. *et al.* (1988) Effects of electrical muscle stimulation combined with voluntary contractions after knee ligament surgery. *Med. Sci. Sports Exerc.*, **20**, 93–98

Wojtys, E.M., Goldstein, S.A., Redfern, M. *et al.* (1987) A biomechanical evaluation of the Lenox Hill knee brace. *Clin. Orthop.*, **220**, 179–184

Woo, S.L.-Y. and Buckwalter, J.A. (eds) (1987) *Injury and Repair of the Musculoskeletal Soft Tissues*, American Academy of Orthopaedic Surgeons, pp. 114–117

Wotjys, E.M., Beaman, D.R., Glover, R.A. *et al.* (1990) Innervation of the human knee joint by substance-P fibres. *Arthroscopy,* **6**, 254–263

Appendix I Stages in recovery after injury

1 Reduce inflammation	Compression Cooling Anti-inflammatory agent
2 Maintain movement	Active assisted exercise Joint and muscle massage Stretching
3 Increase power*	Isometric exercise through a pain-free range Co-contraction of quadriceps and hamstrings Resisted exercise (antigravity, theraband, springs, weights) Closed chain activity
4 Regain fitness	Graded strengthening (closed and open chain) Cardiovascular work (hydrotherapy, jogging, arm ergometer) Progression of sport-specific skills

* Monitor the knee by avoiding the production of effusion and pain.

Appendix II

TEGNER ACTIVITY SCALE

10 Competitive sports
    Soccer – national or international level
 9 Competitive sports
    Soccer – lower divisions
    Ice hockey
    Wrestling
    Gymnastics
 8 Competitive sports
    Bandy
    Squash or badminton
    Athletics (jumping, etc)
    Downhill skiing
 7 Competitive sports
    Tennis
    Athletics (running)
    Motocross or speedway
    Handball or basketball
  Recreational sports
    Soccer
    Bandy or ice hockey
    Squash
    Athletics (jumping)
    Cross-country track finding (orienteering)
    both recreational and competitive
 6 Recreational sports
    Tennis or badminton
    Handball or basketball
    Downhill skiing
    Jogging, at least 5 times weekly
 5 Work
    Heavy labour (e.g. construction, forestry)
  Competitive sports
    Cycling
    Cross-country skiing
  Recreational sports
    Jogging on uneven ground at least twice weekly
 4 Work
    Moderately heavy work (e.g. truck driving, scrubbing floors)

Recreational sports
    Cycling
    Cross-country skiing
    Jogging on even ground at least twice weekly
3 Work
    Light work (e.g. nursing)
Competitive and recreational sports
    Swimming
Walking in rough forest terrain
2 Work
    Light work
Walking on uneven ground
1 Work
    Sedentary work
Walking on even ground
0 Sick leave or disability pension because of knee problems

LYSHOLM KNEE SCORES

Limp	
None	5
Slight or periodic	3
Severe and constant	0
Support	
None	5
Stick or crutch needed	2
Weight bearing impossible	0
Locking	
None	15
Catching sensation, but no locking	10
Locking occasionally	6
Locking frequently	2
Locked joint at examination	0
Instability	
Never	25
Rarely during athletic activities	20
Frequently during athletic activities	15
Occasionally during daily activities	10
Often during daily activities	5
Every step	0
Pain	
None	25
Inconstant and slight during strenuous activities	20
Marked during or after walking more than 2 km	10
Marked during or after walking less than 2 km	5
Constant	0
Swelling	
None	10
After strenuous activities	6

After ordinary activities	3
Constant	0
Stairs	
No problem	10
Slight problem	6
One step at a time	3
Impossible	0
Squatting	
No problem	5
Slight problem	4
Not beyond 90° of flexion of the knee	2
Impossible	0

CINCINNATI KNEE RATING SYSTEM

Symptom rating scale
Normal knee
Strenuous work/sports
    Jumping
    Hard pivoting   10

Moderate work/sports
    Running, turning, twisting
    Symptoms with strenuous work/sports   8

Light work/sports
    No running, twisting jumping
    Symptoms with moderate work/sports   6

Daily living activities
    Symptoms with light work/sports   4
    Moderate symptoms (frequent, limiting)   2
    Severe symptoms (constant, not relieved)   0

Sports activities
Level 1 (participates 4–7 days per week)
    Jumping
    Hard pivoting
    Cutting (basketball, volleyball, football
    gymnastics, soccer)   100

    Running
    Twisting
    Turning (tennis, racquetball, handball
    baseball, ice hockey, field hockey, skiing
    wrestling)   95

    No running, twisting, jumping (cycling, swimming)   90

Level II   (participates 1–3 days per week)
Jumping
Hard pivoting
Cutting (basketball, volleyball, football, gymnastics,
soccer)   85

Running
Twisting
Turning (tennis, racquetball, handball, baseball,
ice hockey, field hockey, skiing, wrestling)   80

No running, twisting, jumping (cycling, swimming)   75

Level III (participates 1–3 times per month)
Jumping
Hard pivoting
Cutting (basketball, volleyball, football, gymnastics,
soccer)   ·65

Running
Twisting
Turning (tennis, racquetball, handball, baseball,
ice hockey, field hockey, skiing, wrestling)   60

No running, twisting, jumping (cycling, swimming)   55

Level IV   Daily living activities (No sports)
Without problems   40
Moderate problems   20
Severe problems – on crutches, full disability   0

ASSESSMENT OF FUNCTION
Walking
Normal, unlimited   40
Some limitations   30
Only 3–4 blocks possible   20
Less than one block, cane, crutch   0

Stair climbing
Normal, unlimited   40
Some limitations   30
Only 11–30 steps possible   20
Only 1–10 steps possible   0

Squatting, kneeling
Normal, unlimited   40
Some limitations   30
Only 6–10 possible   20
Only 0–5 possible   0

Sports
    Straight running
        Fully competitive   100
        Some limitations, guarding   80
        Run half-speed, definite limitations   60
        Not able to do   40

Sports	
Straight running	
Fully competitive	100
Some limitations, guarding	80
Run half-speed, definite limitations	60
Not able to do	40
Jumping/landing on affected leg	
Fully competitive	100
Some limitations	80
Definite limitations, half-speed	60
Not able to do	40
Hard twisting/cutting/pivoting	
Fully competitive	100
Some limitations, guarding	80
Definite limitations, half-speed	60
Not able to do	40

Glossary

Abrasion. A deep grazing of the skin caused by friction; further injury of the underlying soft tissue should always be suspected.

Actin-myosin coupling. The energy-dependent process by which the components of muscle contract.

Aponeurosis. A sheet of thin connective tissue overlying muscle or bone.

Apophysis. A growth centre in juvenile bone at which a musculotendinous unit attaches, and thus a site for traction injuries and 'growing pains'.

Arthralgia. An inflammatory condition of one or more joints, generally secondary to a systemic condition.

Articular. Pertaining to a joint, and in particular to the cartilage surfaces.

Atrophy. Wasting or loss of bulk (and strength).

Axial. Along the line of a limb (the adjective is also used to describe structures composing and linked to the spine).

Axontmesis. A disruption of the axon, causing Wallerian degeneration, but the nerve sheath is preserved.

Blister. A collection of clear fluid (serum) below the superficial layer of the skin caused by repeated friction and the resultant inflammation of the tissues.

Cancellous (metaphyseal) bone. The 'spongy' network of bone which forms the ends of long bones in adults, and which lies between the diaphysis (shaft) and epiphysis of a juvenile long bone; cancellous bone also forms the bulk of discrete bones such as the patella, calcaneum and vertebra.

Compartment syndrome. An increase in tissue pressure within a relatively inelastic fascial space leading to serious neurovascular compromise (see p. 178).

Contraction. The active process of muscle shortening.

Contracture. Adaptive shortening of muscle and connective tissue if a joint ceases to move through its full range; this shrinkage can prove difficult to reverse and must therefore be prevented.

Coronal. The side-to-side plane of the body (right/left).

Cortical bone. Compact, lamellar bone making up the surface and diaphyses (shafts) of the skeleton.

Crepitus. A grating feeling or sound produced either by the fractured ends of bone rubbing against each other or by friction of soft tissue (such as occurs in tenosynovitis or osteoarthritis).

Dislocation. Complete separation of one articular surface from its comrade surface.

Ecchymosis. A deep and widespread discolouration of skin and tissue produced by haemorrhage from a torn ligament, articular injury or fracture.

Epiphyseal plate (the physis). The cartilaginous and very cellular growing end of a young bone, between the metaphysis and the epiphysis.

Fascia. A sheet or band of strong connective tissue, often linking muscle to bone.

Feedback loop. The sensory and motor reflex arc which maintains balance, muscle tone and joint integrity (see p. 2).

Fibrosis. The production of scar tissue as an end-stage of chronic or repeated inflammation; a contracture of a joint or loss of muscle function may result.

Fixed flexion deformity. A loss of joint extension, usually permanent, which has been produced by soft tissue contracture or deformity of bone.

Gait. The walking pattern of an individual, comprised of alternating strides at a particular cadence; gait may be antalgic (painful), short-leg or Trendelenburg (due to abnormal hip mechanics) or altered as a result of a stiff knee.

Glide. Forward-back or side-to-side movement of one joint on another without any pivoting around the fulcrum of the joint; some glide is normal and necessary, but an excess of this movement results from pathological laxity and makes a joint feel unstable.

Haematoma. A deep but localised bruise, generally involving muscle.

Haemophilia. A genetically-determined coagulation disorder, mainly affecting males.

Hyperpathia. Increased and unpleasant perception of sensation, usually pain, in an area where the sensory nerves have been injured and are now recovering.

Hyperpression. A syndrome characterised by excessive pressure of the patella laterally against the lateral femoral condyle.

Hypertrophy. Increased size of muscle fibre or other soft tissue as a result of regular use.

Hypopression. Loss of the normal articulating pressure between joint surfaces (such as the medial patellar facet) which may affect the nutrition of articular cartilage.

Instability. The feeling of weakness or giving way that results from abnormal joint or muscle function.

Isokinetic. A type of contraction or exercise where the resistance applied varies but the speed of movement is constant.

Isometric. A type of contraction or exercise where the speed of movement is held constant but the resistance varies (see above).

Isotonic. A type of contraction or exercise where no movement is made by the limb against a fixed resistance.

Joint lubrication. A process of reducing friction in joints which is dependent upon the fluid-film characteristics of synovial fluid and the biological characteristics of articular cartilage.

Juvenile chronic arthritis. An auto-immune inflammation of one or many joints related to rheumatoid arthritis and previously known as Still's disease.

Kinesiology. The study of motion of the human body and its limbs.

Laxity. Inherited or post-traumatic looseness of a joint owing to ligament incompetence.

Locking. A loss of the extremes of joint movement (see p. 8) as a result of an obstruction between the articular surfaces.

Medial tibial syndrome (junior leg). An adhesive or occasionally a compressive syndrome affecting the lower tibialis posterior muscle and its tendon, principally in young athletes.

Myositis (ossificans). A traumatic, inflammatory condition of muscle which may result in the deposition of calcified tissue in the site of a muscle bleed.

Neuroma. A thickening of the nerve resulting from the sprouting of axons at the site of injury, and the fibrotic nature of the healing process.

Neuropraxia. A temporary interruption of nerve conduction caused by oedema of the axon, but without any break in the continuity of the axon or its sheath.

Neurotmesis. Disruption of both the axon and its sheath resulting in a variable gap between the nerve ends and the formation of a neuroma.

Osteoarthritis. The destruction and ineffectual repair of articular surfaces of a joint produced by abnormal wear, and resulting in stiffness and deformity of the joint.

Osteochondritis dissecans. A pathological process affecting subchondral bone, classically in the medial femoral condyle, which may cause an osteochondral fragment to separate (see p. 167).

Paraestesiase. Abnormal perception of sensation, usually with a painful component.

Patella alta (high patella). A description of the position of the patella in relation to the femoral condylar groove.

Patella baja (low patella). A rare, inferiorly positioned patella.

Pes anserinus ('the goose's foot'). A group of muscles (sartorius, gracilis and semitendinosus) which help to stabilise the medial side of the knee in dynamic fashion and also internally rotate the tibia.

Proprioception. The sense of feeling in a joint or muscle, which depends upon a feedback loop.

Pseudo-locking. A feeling of restricted joint movement, particularly flexion, which is not caused by an intra-articular obstruction (often the result of patellar instability).

Q-angle. The angle between the axis of the pull of the quadriceps muscle (described by a line from the anterior superior iliac spine to the centre of the patella) and the patellar tendon (approximately 10–15 degrees normally).

Quadriceps inhibition. A reflex prevention of quadriceps muscle contraction produced by serious pathology in the knee, mainly as a result of pain and capsular distention.

Recurvatum. Hyperextension or a bending backwards of the knee joint, often seen in those with ligament laxity or following trauma.

Reflex arc. Similar to a feedback loop, comprising afferent and efferent nerves (see p. 2).

Rheumatoid arthritis. An auto-immune systemic disease of connective tissue involving synovial joints and characterised by remissions and exacerbations.

Rotatory instability. A complex instability resulting from abnormal rotation of the femur upon the weightbearing tibia and perceived by the patient as a knee that is not 'true'.

Sagittal. The anteroposterior (forward-back) plane of the body; knee flexion and the drawer tests occur in this plane.

Shin splints. An exercise-induced (and therefore reversible) compartment syndrome involving the anterior compartment of the calf (also used to describe the medial tibial syndrome and tibial stress fracture).

Sprain. A partial tear of a ligament.

Strain. A tear of muscle fibres.

Subluxation. A partial dislocation in which some articular surface contact is still maintained.

Tenosynovitis. An inflammatory condition of a tendon within its synovial sheath, causing pain, crepitus and loss of function.

Tilt. An abnormal angulation of a joint at right angles to its normal plane of movement, and therefore usually in the coronal plane.

Tinel sign. A tingling feeling (paraesthesiae) transmitted down a nerve when the site of an axontmesis is tapped lightly.

Torsion. An axial deformation of a long bone (generally the femur or tibia) or a rotating movement at a joint (better termed rotation or twisting).

Tracking. The normal movement of a structure within a groove or reciprocal surface, such as the patella between the femoral condyles.

Valgus. A lateral deviation of the peripheral segment of the joint (the knock-knee deformity).

Varus. A medial deviation of the peripheral segment of a joint (the bow-leg deformity).

Vascular. Pertaining to blood vessels and the supply of blood to a part of the body.

Wasting. A colloquial term for the atrophy of a muscle secondary to disuse or disease.

Index